教育部、国家语委重大文化工程

　"中华思想文化术语传播工程"成果

国家社科基金重大项目

　"中国核心术语国际影响力研究"（项目号：21&ZD158）成果

中华思想文化术语传播工程

Key Concepts in
Chinese Thought and Culture

李照国　吴青　邢玉瑞　主编

中医文化

关键词 2

汉英对照

-2-

第二版

Key Concepts in
Traditional Chinese Medicine II

(Chinese-English) *2nd Edition*

外语教学与研究出版社
FOREIGN LANGUAGE TEACHING AND RESEARCH PRESS
北京 BEIJING

图书在版编目（CIP）数据

中医文化关键词 . 2：汉英对照 / 李照国，吴青，邢玉瑞主编 . -- 2 版 .
北京：外语教学与研究出版社，2024. 9. -- ISBN 978-7-5213-5649-6

I . R2-61

中国国家版本馆 CIP 数据核字第 2024B2V191 号

出 版 人　王　芳
责任编辑　刘　佳
责任校对　牛茜茜
封面设计　李　高　彩奇风
版式设计　XXL Studio
出版发行　外语教学与研究出版社
社　　址　北京市西三环北路 19 号（100089）
网　　址　https://www.fltrp.com
印　　刷　北京捷迅佳彩印刷有限公司
开　　本　710×1000　1/16
印　　张　20
字　　数　337 千字
版　　次　2024 年 9 月第 2 版
印　　次　2024 年 9 月第 1 次印刷
书　　号　ISBN 978-7-5213-5649-6
定　　价　88.00 元

如有图书采购需求，图书内容或印刷装订等问题，侵权、盗版书籍等线索，请拨打以下电话或关注官方服务号：
客服电话：400 898 7008
官方服务号：微信搜索并关注公众号“外研社官方服务号”
外研社购书网址：https://fltrp.tmall.com

物料号：356490001

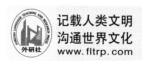

编写委员会

主编： 李照国　吴　青　邢玉瑞

Editors-in-chief: Li Zhaoguo, Wu Qing, Xing Yurui

中文撰稿人： 邢玉瑞　乔文彪

Chinese version: Xing Yurui, QiaoWenbiao

英文翻译： 李照国　吴　青　李晓莉　陈铸芬
　　　　　翟书娟　周阿剑　董　俭

English version: Li Zhaoguo, Wu Qing, Li Xiaoli, Chen Zhufen,
　　　　　　Zhai Shujuan, Zhou Ajian, Dong Jian

出版说明

　　出版于 2018 年 5 月的《中医文化关键词》对精选的 111 条中医思想文化基本术语（主要围绕精、气、阴阳理论、五行和部分与藏象相关的概念）进行了阐释，本辑主要涉及藏象、经络、病因病机和治则治法术语，包括 110 条术语、术语表、索引和参考书目。每条术语包含术语拼音、术语中文、术语英文、术语中文解释、术语英文解释、术语曾经译法（2000 年之前的翻译）、术语现行译法（2000 年之后的翻译）、术语标准译法、翻译说明以及引例。读者通过阅读术语词条，不仅能够了解术语的中文含义以及英文解释，还能够通过比较摘引的"曾经译法"和"现行译法"，结合"翻译说明"，了解中医术语翻译研究近 40 年来的发展变化。同时，书中提供的引例可以帮助读者了解术语在中医典籍中的具体应用。本书采用中英文对照体例，这对想要学习、了解和借鉴中医文化内涵的国内外读者大有裨益，也为读者从事中医药英译、中华文化传播与国际交流以及中医文献研究提供了宝贵的素材。

Note to Readers

Key Concepts in Traditional Chinese Medicine published in May 2018 includes 111 very basic terms concerning the thoughts and culture of traditional Chinese medicine (TCM), mainly related to essence, qi, the theory of yin and yang, five elements, and visceral manifestation. This book covers 110 terms related to visceral manifestation, meridians, etiology, pathogenesis, therapeutic principles and methods, providing simplified Chinese characters, Mandarin pronunciation in pinyin, English translation of each term, definitions in both Chinese and English, previous translation (used before year 2000), current translation (used after year 2000), standard translation, explanatory notes as well as citations from TCM classics in both Chinese and English. A list of concepts, index, and reference books are placed at the very end of the book. It is expected that readers not only understand the Chinese meaning and English translation of the terms but also gain a deeper understanding of the progress made over a period of 40 years in the studies of TCM term translation by comparing their "previous translation" with their "current translation" in combination with the "explanatory notes." In addition, readers can gain an insight into the specific application of the included terms by referring to their corresponding citations. This bilingual book can be a helpful resource to the readers at home and abroad who want to learn, understand, and draw on the fundamental concepts in TCM. It may serve as valuable reference material for the readers who would like to engage in the English translation of TCM texts, the international communication of Chinese culture, and the research on TCM literature.

前　言

中医是中国医药学的简称，是中国特有的一门与天文、地理和人文密切交融的古典医学体系。中医以中国的传统文化、古典哲学和人文思想为理论基础，融合诸子之学和百家之论，综合自然科学和社会科学的理论与实践，构建了独具特色的理论体系、思辨模式和诊疗方法。中医重视人与自然的和谐共处，强调文化传承的一以贯之，提倡人与社会的和谐发展，为各地医药的创建、文化的传播和文明的发展开辟了广阔的路径。这正如2016年国务院颁布的《中国的中医药》白皮书对中医的文化定位，中医是"中华文明的杰出代表"，"对世界文明进步产生了积极影响"，"实现了自然科学与人文科学的融合和统一"，"蕴含了中华民族深邃的哲学思想"。

中医是世界上历史悠久、文化深厚、体系完整、疗效显著、应用广泛、发展迅速的一门传统医学体系。早在先秦时期，中医已经逐步传入朝鲜等周边地区。汉唐时期，中医已经传入日本、东南亚地区。18世纪之后，中医逐步传入欧洲并在19世纪中期得到了较为广泛的传播。20世纪70年代之后，随着针刺麻醉术的研制成功，中医很快传遍全球，为世界医药的发展，为各国民众的健康，为中华文化的传播做出了巨大的贡献。由于理法先进、文化深厚、方药自然、疗效神奇，中医这门古老的医学体系虽历经数千年而始终昌盛不衰，为中华民族的繁衍、为中华文明的发展、为中华文化的传播开辟了独特的蹊径。

中医的四大经典——即《黄帝内经》《难经》《神农本草经》《伤寒杂病论》——不仅代表着中医最为核心的理论和方法，而且还代表着中华文化最为核心的思想和精神，特别是《黄帝内经》，几乎涉及中国古代自然科学、社会科学和语言文化等各个方面，其在世界各地的传播已经成为中国文化走向世界的康庄大道。阴（yin）、阳（yang）、气（qi）等中国文化重要概念的音译形式已经成为西方语言中的通用语，这就是中医为中国文化走出去做出的一大贡献，为中国文化走出去奠定了坚实的语言基础。

中国文化要西传，要走向世界，自然需要有一个各国学术领域、文化领域和民间人士所关注的方面，借以引导各界人士关注中国文化。汉唐时期西域佛界人士千里迢迢到中原地区宣扬佛教，明清时期西方传教士远渡重洋到中国传播基督教，医药一直是他们凝聚人心和人力的一个重要的路径。作为中国传统文化不可分割的一个重要组成部分，中医对于推进中国文化走向世界，不仅是凝聚异国他乡人心和人力的一个重要渠道，而且还是直接传播和传扬中国传统文化的一个重要桥梁。任何一位想要学习、了解和借鉴中医理法方药的外国人士，首先必须要学习和掌握阴阳学说、五行学说和精气学说等中国传统文化的基本理论和思想，这已经成为国际间的一个共识。

由此可见，要使中国文化全面、系统地走向世界并为世界各国越来越多人士心诚意正地理解和接受，中医的对外传播无疑是一个最为理想而独特的坚实桥梁。

Preface

TCM, short for traditional Chinese medicine, is a classical medical system with Chinese characteristics that are closely integrated with astronomy, geography, and humanities. Based on traditional Chinese culture, classical philosophy and humanistic thoughts, TCM, in combination with the various schools of thought and their exponents during the period from pre-Qin times to the early years of the Han Dynasty as well as the theories and practice of natural sciences and social sciences, constitutes the unique theoretical system, way of thinking as well as diagnosis and treatment methods. TCM has a high regard for the harmonious coexistence of man and nature. It emphasizes consistent cultural inheritance, advocates the harmonious development between man and society, and opens broad prospects for local medicine development, cultural dissemination, and the progress of human civilization. As promulgated in the white paper "Traditional Chinese Medicine in China" by the State Council in 2016, TCM is a "representative feature of Chinese civilization," which "produces a positive impact on the progress of human civilization," "represents a combination of natural sciences and humanities," and "embraces profound philosophical ideas of the Chinese nation."

TCM is a comprehensive and widely used traditional medical system in the world with a long history. It is characterized by profound culture, distinctive effects, and rapid development. Early in the pre-Qin period, TCM had been gradually introduced into the neighboring areas such as the Korean Peninsula. During the Han and Tang dynasties, it had been brought into Japan and Southeast Asia. After the eighteenth century, TCM was introduced into Europe and it gained wide dissemination in the mid-nineteenth century. After the 1970s, TCM quickly spread all over the world along with the success of acupuncture anesthesia, contributing substantially to the development of world medicine, the wellbeing of all nations and the dissemination of Chinese culture. Due to its advanced theory, profound cultural basis, natural therapy, and remarkable effectiveness, TCM has survived and prospered throughout the ages. It has blazed a unique path for the prosperity of the Chinese nation, the development of Chinese civilization, and the spread of Chinese culture.

Four TCM classics—*Yellow Emperor's Internal Canon of Medicine, Canon of Difficult Issues, Agriculture God's Canon of Materia Medica*, and *Treatise on Cold Damage and Miscellaneous Diseases*—not only represent the core of TCM theory and method but also contain the essence of thought and spirit in Chinese culture, among which *Yellow Emperor's Internal Canon of Medicine* is the landmark. It involves almost every aspect of natural sciences, social sciences as well as language and culture in ancient China. Its worldwide spread has become a great way for Chinese culture to go global. The transliteration form of the important concepts of Chinese culture such as yin, yang and qi has been adopted in Western languages. This is a great contribution made by TCM to the "going out" of Chinese culture, and it has laid a solid language foundation for Chinese culture going out.

Chinese culture is going to spread to the West, to the world. Naturally, there is a need for attention from various academic, cultural, and civil sectors. In the Han and Tang dynasties, the Buddhists in Xiyu (the Western regions) travelled all the way to Central China to promote Buddhism whereas in the Ming and Qing dynasties Western missionaries worked their way to China to spread Christianity. For both of them, medicine has been an important means to rally public support. As an integral part of traditional Chinese culture, TCM not only plays an important role in rallying foreign support to stimulate Chinese culture to go global but also serves as a bridge to disseminate and promote traditional Chinese culture directly. It is an international consensus that anyone desiring to learn, understand, and draw on TCM theories, methods, formulas, and herbs shall first of all learn and acquire the basic theories and thoughts of traditional Chinese culture, for example, the theory of yin and yang, the theory of five elements, and the theory of essence and qi.

It can be seen that the international communication of TCM is undoubtedly an ideal, unique, and solid approach if Chinese culture is to go global in a comprehensive and systematic manner and to gain the heartfelt understanding and acceptance from the people worldwide.

目 录
Contents

tiān rén héyī

天人合一

Oneness of Heaven and Human

中国古代关于天与人、天道与人道、自然与人为相统一的思想。天人合一作为中国古代哲学的重要命题，在不同的历史时期有不同的含义。从中医学的角度而言，主要反映为一是人与自然同源，即宇宙万物和人均由元气生成；二是人与自然同构，即宇宙万物和人具有元气、阴阳、五行等相同的结构；三是人与自然同道，即人与自然万物之间具有相同的阴阳消长及五行生克制化规律。

天人合一观作为中国传统文化的核心思想，把天地宇宙确定为人存在的境域，规定了人的物性、存在价值取向、人生境界和超越维度以及认识方式与思维方式。中医学借用和发挥了天人合一的哲学观，以此作为自己的认识论、方法论和价值观，来建构中医理论体系并指导中医临床实践。

The term refers to a concept in traditional Chinese thought, i.e., the unity between heaven and human, between the way of heaven and the way of human, and between nature and human. It is an important proposition of ancient Chinese philosophy with its varied meanings in different historical contexts. From the perspective of traditional Chinese medicine (TCM), it mainly denotes that man and nature are homologous, i.e., all things in the universe including human beings are derived from original qi. In addition, man and nature are isomorphic, i.e., all things in the universe including human beings are of the same structure composed of original qi, yin, yang, and the five elements, etc. Finally, man and nature follow identical laws, i.e., man and nature observe similar principles of waxing and waning of yin and yang as well as the principles of generation, restriction, inhibition, and transformation among the five elements.

As the core of traditional Chinese culture, the concept of heaven-human oneness defines the universe as the realm of human existence; thus, it stipulates the physical attributes, the value orientation, the realm of life, and the dimension of transcendence as well as the way of understanding and thinking of human beings. This concept is then borrowed and further developed as the epistemology, methodology, and value system for the construction of theoretical system and the guidance of clinical practice of TCM.

【曾经译法】 unite the nature with human being; Human body corresponds to the nature

【现行译法】 unity of the heaven and humanity; holistic view of the heaven and environment

【标准译法】 oneness of heaven and human

【翻译说明】 译词 oneness 表示"一体；一致；和谐"，比 unity（统一体；联合体；整体）更能体现"合一"之意。译词 humanity 偏于强调"人类；人性；人文；人道"。"天人"译为 heaven and human 可构成押头韵。

引例 Citations:

◎人与天地相参也，与日月相应也。（《灵枢·岁露论》）

（人与天地自然相参证，与日月运转相应合。）

Man follows the laws of nature, and corresponds to the working principles of the sun and the moon. (*Spiritual Pivot*)

◎人以天地之气生，四时之法成。（《素问·宝命全形论》）

（人依靠天地之气来生存，随着四时变化规律而成长。）

Man depends on the heaven qi and the earth qi for existence and lives in accordance with the principle of the four seasons. (*Plain Conversation*)

◎儒者则因明致诚，因诚致明，故天人合一，致学而可以成圣，得天而未始遗人。（《正蒙·乾称篇》）

（儒者则由明察人伦而通达天理之诚，由通达天理之诚而洞明世事，因此天与人相合为一，通过学习而可以成为圣人，把握天理而不曾遗失对人伦的洞察。）

Confucianists, on the other hand, have a clear understanding of the heavenly principle by observing human relations, and thus understand worldly affairs by referring to the heavenly principle. Therefore, man and heaven are united in oneness. Men can become sages through learning, having both a command of the heavenly principle and an insight into human relations. (*Enlightenment Through Confucian Teachings*) xíng shén yītǐ

形神一体

Unity of Body and Spirit

形神一体是中国古代哲学与中医学有关生理与心理关系的重要命题。形，指形体，即脏腑身形；神，指以五神、五志为特征的心理活动。中医学认为人的形体与精神，是一个不可分割的统一整体，神由形而生，神依形而存，神寓于形中，形盛则神旺，形衰则神去，二者相伴相随，俱生俱灭。《素问·上古天真论》把这种关系概括为"形与神俱"，确立了唯物主义的形神观念。在肯定形体决定精神的同时，又十分强调神对形的主宰作用，认为人体脏腑功能的协调，对外界自然、社会环境的适应，均离不开神的调节作用。

The term refers to an important proposition of ancient Chinese philosophy and traditional Chinese medicine (TCM) concerning the relationship between physiology and psychology. "Body" refers to the physical aspect, i.e., zang-fu organs and physical form; "spirit" refers to the spiritual aspect, i.e., mental activities characterized by the five spirits and the five emotions. In TCM, body and spirit are an inseparable unity. They go hand in hand to flourish alike or to perish together. Spirit is born from and dependent on physical body for existence. Residing in physical body, spirit will be vigorous when one is physically abundant and exhaustive when one is physically diminished. Their relationship was summarized in the section "Discussion on Ancient Innocence Theory" of *Plain Conversation* as the "harmony between body and spirit," which marked the establishment of the materialist concept of body and spirit. While affirming the physical body determines spirit, it also emphasizes the dominance of spirit over body. It is believed that the coordination of the functions of the zang-fu organs and their adaptation to the external natural and social environments are inseparable from the regulation of spirit.

【曾经译法】 unity of body and spirit

【现行译法】unity of physique and spirit; unity of body and spirit; integration of body and spirit

【标准译法】unity of body and spirit

【翻译说明】"形神一体"指人的形体与精神是一个不可分割的统一整体，故而译作 unity of body and spirit。相对而言，译词 physique 强调形体的大小、强弱，integration 常用来表示结合、融合之意，与术语含义略有出入。

引例 Citations:

◎故能形与神俱，而尽终其天年，度百岁乃去。(《素问·上古天真论》)

（所以能够使形体与精神和谐统一，并存无损，从而享尽天年，活到百岁才离开人世。）

That is why they could maintain harmony and unity of body and spirit, enjoying good health and long life. (*Plain Conversation*)

◎形者神之体，神者形之用。无神则形不可活，无形则神无以生。(《类经·针刺类》)

（形是神存在的载体，神是形的生命体现。没有了神则形体不能存活，没有了形体则神无以生成。）

Form is the vehicle for spirit, and spirit is the embodiment of form. Without spirit, form is lifeless; without form, spirit shall not come into being. (*Classified Classics*)

君主之官

Monarch

国家元首之职。中医认为心主神志，具有主宰人体心理活动和人体脏腑组织器官生理活动的功能。一方面，心是人体心理活动的主宰，对各种心理活动起着整体调节作用，所谓"心为五脏六腑之大主，而总统魂魄，并赅意志"（《类经·疾病类》）；另一方面，人体各脏腑器官的生理功能不同，必须在心的主宰和调节下，才能相互配合，共同完成整体生命活动。正由于心具有主宰人体整个生命活动的功能，故《素问·灵兰秘典论》将心比喻为"君主之官"。

The term refers to a ruler running an empire. In traditional Chinese medicine, the heart governs the mental activity as well as the physiological activities of all organs and tissues in humans. For one thing, the heart governs the mind and regulates various mental activities. As stated in the section "Diseases" of *Classified Classics*, "the heart, being the monarch of the five zang-organs and six fu-organs, commands ethereal soul and corporeal soul, and involves will." For another, it is vital for the heart to coordinate different physiological functions of all organs for the fulfillment of overall life activities. The heart performs the function of governing all human life activities, hence the metaphorical term used in the section "Discussion on the Secret Canons Stored in Royal Library" of *Plain Conversation*.

【曾经译法】 Office of monarch; Heart; monarch organ; organ as monarch

【现行译法】 monarch organ; monarch-organ; king-organ; key organ; heart, which is the organ similar to the monarch

【标准译法】 monarch

【翻译说明】 术语中的"官"指"官职"。该术语翻译主要分为直译和意译。"心"在五脏中的地位犹如"君主"，直译为 monarch，意译为"心脏，heart"。在准确传达中医文化内涵的前提下，首选直译，译为 monarch 不仅体现了"心"在主宰人体整个生命活动中的重要作用，更能传达中医术语命名的文化层面的含义。

引例 Citations:

◎心者一身之主，故为君主之官。(《内经知要》)

(心为全身生命活动的主宰，所以比喻为君主。)

The heart governs the life activities of the whole body, so its role is likened to that of a monarch. (*Essentials of the Internal Canon of Medicine*)

◎君者，人之主也。若以十二脏论之，则心者君主之官也。(《黄帝素问直解》)

(君王是人的主宰。如果以十二脏的关系而论，则心在诸脏中为君主之官。)

The monarch is the ruler of a state. As far as the twelve zang-fu organs are concerned, the heart is regarded as the monarch. (*Direct Interpretation of Plain Conversation in Yellow Emperor's Internal Canon of Medicine*) xiàngfù zhī guān

相傅之官

Prime Minister

相国、宰相、太傅、少傅等辅助君主而治国的官职。中医认为肺具有主气、宣发肃降、朝百脉，协助心脏完成调节全身功能活动的作用，犹如辅佐君主治理国家的宰相一样，故《素问·灵兰秘典论》将肺比喻为"相傅之官"。具体体现在以下几个方面：一是肺司有节奏的呼吸吐纳活动，主持呼吸节律，并以此调节着宗气、营卫之气等的生成。二是肺的宣肃吐纳调节着气机的升降出入，一身脏腑及经络之气、宗气、营卫之气的运动，均是在肺宣发肃降的作用下，实现其正常的升降出入运动。三是肺主气，推动和调节血液的运行，并参与心律、心率的调控。四是肺主宣发肃降，调节机体津液的输布和排泄。

The term refers to the official position of a prime minister, or honored ministers such as *taifu* (太傅, literally grandmaster) and *shaofu* (少傅, literally junior master) who assist the monarch in governing the empire. According to traditional Chinese medicine, the lung governs qi and its dispersion, depuration, as well as descent. Besides, the lung is where all meridians and vessels converge. With these functions, it assists the heart in regulating the functional activities of the whole body in the same manner that the prime minister assists the monarch in governing the empire. Hence the role of the lung is likened to that of the prime minister according to the section "Discussion on the Secret Canons Stored in Royal Library" of *Plain Conversation*. Specifically, the lung is involved in the following functions. First, the lung governs rhythmical respiration, controls the rhythm of breathing, and therefore regulates the generation of pectoral qi, nutrient qi, and defense qi. Second, through dispersion, depuration, and descent, the lung regulates the ascending, descending, exiting, and entering of qi, including the qi in zang-fu organs and meridians, pectoral qi, nutrient qi, and defense qi. Third, the lung governs qi, through which it promotes and regulates blood circulation, and helps to maintain normal heart rhythm and heart rate. Fourth, the lung governs dispersion, depuration, and descent of qi, through which it regulates the distribution and excretion of body fluids.

【曾经译法】 lung

【现行译法】 official acting as the prime minister

【标准译法】 prime minister

【翻译说明】 该术语翻译主要分为直译和意译。"肺"在五脏中的地位犹如"相国、宰相",直译为 prime minister,意译为"肺,lung"。在准确传达中医文化内涵的前提下,首选直译更能传达中医术语命名的文化层面的含义。

引例 Citations:

◎肺与心皆居膈上,位高近君,犹之宰辅,故称相傅之官。(《类经·藏象类》)

（肺与心都位于胸膈以上,位置高而接近君主之官"心",犹如宰相,所以称为相傅之官。）

Both the lung and the heart are in the chest and above the diaphragm. The lung is positioned high, close to the heart—the monarch. It is likened to the prime minister, hence the metaphorical name. (*Classified Classics*)

◎肺为华盖之脏,相傅之官,藏魄而主气者也。(《神农本草经疏》)

（肺为人体上部如伞盖样的脏,犹如宰相,藏魄而主宰一身之气。）

The lung is positioned high in the human body like a "florid canopy." It is likened to the prime minister, housing corporeal soul and governing the qi in the whole body. (*Commentary on the "Agriculture God's Canon of Materia Medica"*) jiāngjūn zhī guān

将军之官

General

　　将军，即高级军事将帅。《素问·灵兰秘典论》比喻人体肝具有运筹帷幄，智勇兼备的特性，犹如高级军事将帅。肝为刚脏，喜条达而恶抑郁，其气易亢，与将军的刚直、勇猛相似；肝主疏泄，调畅情志，参与心神活动，同时肝主少阳春生之气，具有无限生机，故人体计谋、筹划等精神活动由肝主管。若肝失谋虑，常表现为谋略不足，智力障碍，言行迟钝，或有勇无谋，烦躁易怒，甚至发狂等症状。

The term refers to a high rank of officer in the army. As described in the section "Discussion on the Secret Canons Stored in Royal Library" of *Plain Conversation*, it is a metaphor, indicating the role of the liver is likened to that of a senior military commander-in-chief, devising strategies with bravery and wisdom. The liver is the unyielding zang-organ, which prefers free activity and detests depression. Its qi easily becomes hyperactive, like the general being righteous and bold. The liver governs the coursing of qi, regulates emotions, and is involved in mental activities. It corresponds to *shaoyang* upward-rising spring qi, thus full of vitality. Consequently, the liver governs such mental activities as planning and strategizing. If the liver fails to govern planning, such symptoms will occur as poor sense of strategy, retardation, being slow in words and deeds, foolhardiness, vexation, irritability, or even madness.

【曾经译法】 liver; general organ; organ as general

【现行译法】 general-like organ (liver)

【标准译法】 general

【翻译说明】 翻译该术语的方法主要有直译和意译两种。肝喜条达，其气易亢，为刚脏，犹如"将军"，直译为 general，意译为"肝，liver"。在准确传达中医文化内涵的前提下，首选直译更能传达中医术语命名的文化层面的含义。

引例 Citations:

◎勇而能断，故曰将军。(《黄帝内经素问》王冰注)

　　(勇敢而且能够决断，所以称为将军。)

It is brave and decisive, hence the name general. (*Plain Conversation in Yellow Emperor's Internal Canon of Medicine* Annotated by Wang Bing)

◎肝主怒，拟其似者，故曰将军，怒则不复有谋虑，是肝之病也。从病之失职，以测不病时之本能，故谋虑归诸肝。(《群经见智录》)

　　(肝主宰怒的情绪，仿照与它相似的事物，称之为将军。愤怒的情况下，人就不能正常地思考谋划，这是肝的疾病。从疾病情况下的失职，去推测正常时的职能，所以谋虑归属于肝。)

The liver governs anger. It is so named as the general officer by analogy. When people are angry, they lose the ability to plan well, which is a manifestation of the liver disorder. Therefore, in consideration of the symptoms that occur from dysfunction, the liver is believed to govern strategy-making when it functions properly. (*Record of Wisdom Observed in the Medical Classics*) cānglǐn zhī guān

仓廪之官

Granary Officer

管理粮食仓库的官吏。比喻脾胃受纳、运化饮食，化生精微物质的功能。胃主受纳腐熟，脾主运化，脾与胃在功能上密切相关，二者相互配合，人体摄入的饮食物经过胃的腐熟、消化，再经过脾的运化，转化为精气、血、津液，以输送到全身，营养五脏六腑、四肢百骸，犹如粮仓提供给人类粮食一样，所以《素问·灵兰秘典论》称其为"仓廪之官"。若脾胃功能旺盛，则人体营养物质来源充足；否则，精气、血、津液生成不足，就会出现神疲乏力，少气懒言，头晕眼花，消瘦等病症。

The term refers to the official in charge of the granary. It is a metaphor for the functions of the spleen and the stomach in taking in and transporting food and drinks as well as transforming them into essence. Specifically, the stomach receives, stores, and decomposes food, while the spleen governs transportation and transformation. Their functions are closely associated with each other. They cooperate: the ingested food and drinks are decomposed by the stomach, then transported and transformed by the spleen into essential qi, blood, and body fluids before being further transmitted to the whole body to nourish the five zang-organs, six fu-organs, limbs, and bones. The spleen and the stomach work in the same way that a granary provides man with food; hence comes the metaphorical name in the section "Discussion on the Secret Canons Stored in Royal Library" of *Plain Conversation*. If the functions of the spleen and the stomach are vigorous, sources of nutrients will be abundant; otherwise, the generation of essential qi, blood, and body fluids will be insufficient, and symptoms such as lassitude, fatigue, shortness of breath, no desire to speak, dizziness, as well as emaciation can occur.

【曾经译法】 office of the granary (referring to the spleen and stomach); SPLEEN AND STOMACH ARE THE WARE-HOUSE; official of the granaries; barn official; barn organ; spleen and stomach

【现行译法】barn organ; barn official (spleen and stomach); organ of granary

【标准译法】granary officer

【翻译说明】译词 granary 指谷物贮藏所，谷仓；barn 源自古英语，表示存放大麦的房屋，现在既可表示（农家的）仓库，也可表示牛舍，马厩，粮秣房。两者相较，选择 granary。故"仓廪之官"译为 granary officer。

引例 Citations:

◎脾主运化，胃司受纳，通主水谷，故皆为仓廪之官。(《类经·藏象类》)

（脾主管运化水谷，胃主管接纳水谷，二者都主管水谷，所以皆称为仓廪之官。）

The spleen governs the transportation and transformation of food and drinks, and the stomach receives them. Both are in charge, so the spleen and the stomach are described as granary officers. (*Classified Classics*)

◎脾……仓廪之本，营之居也……其华在唇四白，其充在肌。(《素问·六节藏象论》)

（脾……是水谷所藏的根本，是营气所生成的地方……其荣华表现在口唇四周，其功用是充实肌肉。）

The spleen … is the root of the granary which stores food and drinks and is the place where nutrient qi is generated… Spleen manifests its splendor in the lips, and it helps to strengthen muscles. (*Plain Conversation*)

作强之官

Labor Officer

主管人体强力劳作之职的官吏。肾藏精，主发育与生殖，精能够生髓，一方面髓充养骨骼，若肾精充盛，则骨骼坚固，体健力强，动作轻劲多力；另一方面，髓充养脑，脑为髓海，若肾精充盛，则髓海盈满，元神得养，则聪明而多智巧。所以《素问·灵兰秘典论》将肾称为"作强之官，伎巧出焉"。如果不注意养生，纵欲过度，耗伤肾精，骨骼与髓海失其所养，则会导致腰膝酸软，四肢倦怠乏力，甚至头昏、耳鸣，记忆力减退等症状。

The term refers to the official in charge of work requiring laborious efforts (such as building and handicraft making). The kidney stores essence as well as governs growth, development, and reproduction. The essence generates marrow whose functions are two-fold. On the one hand, the marrow nourishes bones. If the kidney essence is abundant, one has strong bones and physical strength, with light but forceful movements. On the other hand, the marrow helps nourish brain—the sea of marrows. If kidney essence is abundant, the sea of marrow will be full and the original spirit will be nourished, then one will be smart, witty, and skillful. Therefore, the kidney was described as the "labor officer and it is responsible for skills" in the section "Discussion on the Secret Canons Stored in Royal Library" of *Plain Conversation*. If little attention is paid to health preservation, e.g., sexual overindulgence, kidney-essence depletion might occur, in which case the bones and marrow will be deprived of nourishment, causing such symptoms as soreness and weakness of waist and knees, weak limbs, fatigue, dizziness, tinnitus, and even memory loss.

【曾经译法】office of labor; kidney

【现行译法】the organ in charge of agility; kidney

【标准译法】labor officer

【翻译说明】此处"官"指官职、官吏，译为 officer 较妥，而不是 office 或者 organ。译词 agility 表示灵活、机敏，不符"作强"（人体强力劳作）之意。故"作强之官"译为 labor officer。

引例 Citations:

◎肾属水而藏精，精为有形之本，精盛形成则作用强，故为作强之官。（《类经·藏象类》）

（肾属水而贮藏精气，精气为人体之根本，精气旺盛形体发育成熟，则形体功能强健，所以称为作强之官。）

The kidney pertains to water. It stores essence which forms the foundation of the human body. When essence becomes abundant and the body matures, body function and physical health are well kept, hence the metaphorical name labor officer. (*Classified Classics*)

◎肾处北方而主骨，宜为作强之官。水能化生万物，故曰伎巧出焉。（《内经知要》）

（肾在五行属水配北方，主人体骨骼，适宜称为"作强之官"。水能够化生万物，所以说"伎巧出焉"。）

The kidney pertains to water according to the five-element theory and corresponds to north. It governs bones, and is named as "labor officer." Water is believed to transform and generate all things, hence the saying "the kidney is responsible for skills." (*Essentials of the Internal Canon of Medicine*) zhōngzhèng zhī guān

中正之官

Justice Officer

中正，不偏不倚、公正之意。胆从位置而言，居于脏腑之中间，其经脉在半表半里之处，如易卦二、五爻的"得中"之位，故称"中"；又因胆内藏精汁，参与人体神的活动，属于奇恒之腑，又属于六腑，泻而不藏，阴阳之性俱禀，藏泻之功并兼，如易卦之"当位""得正"爻，故称为"正"；肝与胆相互为用，肝主谋虑，胆主决断，以做出正确的判断，故《素问·灵兰秘典论》称胆为"中正之官"。若胆气虚怯之人，胆的决断功能失常，则易于出现胆怯易惊、善恐、失眠、多梦等精神情志异常的病变。

Zhongzheng (中正, literally middle and rightness) means fairness, and impartiality. The gallbladder is situated in the middle of the zang-fu organs, and its meridian is located in the half exterior and the half interior, like the "middle" position of the second or the fifth line in a *Yi* hexagram, hence called *zhong* (中, middle). In addition, the gallbladder stores bile and is involved in the mental activities. It is both an extraordinary organ and one of the six fu-organs characterized by discharge without storage. The gallbladder has the attributes of both yin and yang, with dual functions of storage and discharge, like the yang lines in the yang position (the first, third, or fifth line) or the yin lines in the yin position (the second, fourth, or six line) in a *Yi* hexagram, hence called *zheng* (正, rightness or exactness). The liver and the gallbladder are closely connected in functions: the former governs strategy-making and the latter controls decision-making in order to make a sound judgment; hence comes the name "justice officer" in the section "Discussion on the Secret Canons Stored in Royal Library" of *Plain Conversation*. If the gallbladder qi is weak, gallbladder dysfunction occurs in terms of decision-making. As a result, mental and emotional disorders such as timidity, fright, fear, insomnia, and dreaminess may occur.

【曾经译法】official acting as a mediator; office of justice; gallbladder

【现行译法】 the official acting as a mediator; gallbladder; fu-viscera with decisive character

【标准译法】 justice officer

【翻译说明】 译词 mediator 表示调停者、调解人，与“胆主决断，以做出正确的判断”意思不吻合；justice 表示公平、公正，英文释义为 the quality of being fair or reasonable，符合文意。本着术语简洁性和一致性原则，将“中正之官”译为 justice officer。

引例 Citations:

◎刚正果决，直而不疑，故为中正之官。(《黄帝内经素问吴注》)

（刚正而坚决果断，正直而不猜疑，所以称为中正之官。）

It is upright and resolute, honest and assertive, hence the metaphorical name justice officer. (*Plain Conversation in Yellow Emperor's Internal Canon of Medicine Annotated by Wu Kun*)

◎按《六节藏象论》曰：凡十一脏取决于胆也。是诸脏腑各有一定之司，而胆则总揽众职，而决其是非，断其犹豫，不偏不倚，故官名中正。(《素问经注节解》)

（按《六节藏象论》说：凡十一脏功能的发挥，都取决于胆的功能正常。这是说人体各脏腑都有各自的功能，而胆对各脏腑都有调节作用，判断其是非，决断其犹豫，不偏不倚，所以说胆的官名为中正。）

According to the "Discussion on Six-plus-six System and the Manifestations of the Viscera" in *Plain Conversation*, all functions of eleven zang-fu organs depend on the normal function of the gallbladder, which means each of the zang-fu organs has its respective functions, and the gallbladder regulates them, judging right from wrong, making impartial decisions, hence the saying "the gallbladder is the justice officer." (*Adapted Interpretation of Plain Conversation in Yellow Emperor's Internal Canon of Medicine*) zhōudū zhī guān

州都之官

Reservoir Officer

州都，本义为水中可居之处，此作水液汇聚之处理解，比喻膀胱主管水液聚集与外泄的作用。人体脏腑代谢后所形成的津液下输于膀胱，在肾的气化作用下，升清降浊，其清者蒸化升腾，再经过三焦而输布全身，其浊者化为尿液，亦在肾的气化作用下，从尿道排出。清代唐容川《血证论·脏腑病机论》还认为："经所谓气化则能出者，谓膀胱之气，载津液上行外达，出而为汗……"说明水液的排出，包括出汗与排尿都与膀胱的气化作用有关，故《素问·灵兰秘典论》称膀胱为"州都之官，津液藏焉，气化则能出矣"。

Originally *zhoudu* (州都, literally state and capital) refers to a habitable place in the water. Here it is a metaphor for the role of the urinary bladder in governing the storage and discharge of water. The body fluids as a result of metabolism are transmitted to the urinary bladder. With kidney's function of qi transformation, the lucidity ascends and the turbidity descends. The lucid is vaporized and then transmitted to the whole body through triple energizer; the turbid is transformed into urine and then discharged from the urethra. According to the section "Discussion on Zang-fu Pathogenesis" of *Treatise on Blood Syndromes* written by Tang Rongchuan in the Qing Dynasty (1616-1911), "*Yellow Emperor's Internal Canon of Medicine* says that as a result of the qi transformation of the urinary bladder, water is discharged and carried upward and outward, which is manifested as sweat…" This indicates that the discharge of water including sweat and urine is related to the qi-transformation function of the urinary bladder, hence the quotation "the urinary bladder is the reservoir officer and is responsible for storing and discharging water by means of qi transformation" in the section "Discussion on the Secret Canons Stored in Royal Library" of *Plain Conversation*.

【曾经译法】THE OFFICIAL MANAGING THE RESERVOIR; river island

official; Regional Rectifier; bladder

【现行译法】bladder

【标准译法】reservoir officer

【翻译说明】译词 rectifier 表示整流器或纠正者，不符合上下文文意。"膀胱"的对应译文是 urinary bladder。"州都"可理解为水液汇聚之处。本着术语简洁性和一致性原则，将"州都之官"译为 reservoir officer。

引例 Citations:

◎膀胱为水腑，乃水液都会之处，故为州都之官。(《黄帝内经素问集注》)

（膀胱为主水之腑，是水液汇聚的地方，所以称为州都之官。）

The urinary bladder governs water and is the place where the fluids are stored, hence the name reservoir officer. (*Collective Annotations of Plain Conversation in Yellow Emperor's Internal Canon of Medicine*)

◎膀胱位居最下，三焦水液所归，是同都会之地，故曰州都之官，津液藏焉。(《类经·藏象类》)

（膀胱位居腹腔最下部，三焦的水液汇集之地，这如同都会之地，所以称为州都之官，津液藏于这里。）

The urinary bladder is at the bottom of the abdominal cavity where the water in triple energizer gathers, like a reservoir. Hence it is named reservoir officer, responsible for storing fluids. (*Classified Classics*) chuándào zhī guān

传道之官

Transportation Officer

比喻大肠犹如负责转运物品的官员。大肠包括结肠和直肠，其上端在阑门处与小肠相接，下端连肛门。大肠接纳小肠下注的消化物，吸收剩余的水分和养料，使糟粕形成粪便，传送至肛门排出体外。大肠的主要生理功能是传导糟粕，故《素问·灵兰秘典论》称之为"传道之官"。大肠转化糟粕的功能失常，主要表现为排便的异常，常见大便秘结或泄泻。

The large intestine is likened to an official in charge of transporting goods. It, including the sigmoid colon and the rectum, joins the small intestine at the ileocolic opening and ends at the anus. Receiving the undigested substances from the small intestine, the large intestine is primarily involved in the absorption of water and nutrients from food residues, forming feces, and defecation. It is this important function of transporting the waste substances that gives it the name transportation officer, which was written in the section "Discussion on the Secret Canons Stored in Royal Library" of *Plain Conversation*. Disorders such as constipation or diarrhea are commonly reported if the large intestine fails to perform its transportation task.

【曾经译法】 official in charge of transportation (large intestine); official in charge of transportation; transportation official; office of conveyance; organ with the function of transmission

【现行译法】 the organ in charge of transportation; organ in charge of transmission; transportation organ (large intestine); organ responsible for conveyance; official of transportation; officer in charge of transportation

【标准译法】 transportation officer

【翻译说明】 "传道之官"比喻大肠犹如负责转运物品的官员。译词

transportation 表示通过道路、交通工具等把人、货物等从一个地方运送到另一个地方；conveyance 侧重运送的过程，也可表示车辆等运载工具；transmission 表示传送、传递、传输、传染、发送（电子信号）等意思。相较而言，transportation 更符合文意。按照术语简洁性和一致性原则，将"传道之官"译为 transportation officer。

引例 Citations:

◎大肠居小肠之下，主出糟粕，是名变化传道。（《内经知要》）

（大肠位置在小肠之下，主要功能是排出糟粕，这就是变化、传道。）

The large intestine starts from the terminal point of the small intestine. Its primary function includes the removal of waste substances, which involves conversion and transportation. (*Essentials of the Internal Canon of Medicine*)

◎大肠所以能传道者，以其为肺之腑，肺气下达，故能传道，是以理大便必须调肺气也。（《中西汇通医经精义》）

（大肠所以能够传导糟粕的原因，是大肠为与肺相配合的腑，肺气下降，所以能够传导糟粕，故调理大便必须调理肺气。）

The reason why the large intestine can transport waste substances is that it is closely related to the lung. The lung governs descent of qi, so the large intestine can transport wastes. Hence it is necessary to regulate lung qi for the regulation of defecation. (*Essentials of Integrated Traditional Chinese and Western Medicine*) juédú zhī guān

决渎之官

Drainage Officer

负责疏通水道的官员。比喻三焦具有疏通水道、运行水液的功能。人体水液的输布和排泄，是由肺、脾、肾等脏的协同作用来完成的，但必须以三焦为通道，以三焦通行元气为动力，才能正常地升降出入运行。若三焦水道不利，则肺、脾、肾等脏调节水液代谢的功能也难以实现，从而出现尿少、水肿等病变。故《素问·灵兰秘典论》曰："三焦者，决渎之官，水道出焉。"

The term refers to the official responsible for dredging waterways, meaning the job of triple energizer is to dredge water passage and transport water. The distribution and excretion of human body fluids is completed through the synergistic function of different organs including the lung, the spleen, and the kidney, which is only made possible when triple energizer serves as the water passage and its qi serves as the driving force. If triple energizer fails to perform its function, it becomes difficult for the lung, the spleen, and the kidney to regulate water metabolism, which may result in less urine, edema, and other pathological changes. According to the section "Discussion on the Secret Canons Stored in Royal Library" of *Plain Conversation*, "triple energizer is the drainage officer and is responsible for regulating the pathway for water transport in the whole body."

【曾经译法】the official who manages the dredging of water (triple warmer); the official managing the dredging of water pathway; the irrigation official who builds waterways; water-course dredging official; organ for water excretion

【现行译法】the organ in charge of water circulation; organ in charge of water drainage (triple energizer); organ for water excretion; triple energizer

【标准译法】drainage officer

【翻译说明】"决渎"表示疏通水道。译词 dredge 表示 to remove mud, stones, etc. from the bottom of a river, canal, etc. using a boat or special machine, to make it deeper or to search for something，强调疏浚、清淤；drainage 表示排水，英文释义为 the system or process by which water or other liquids are drained from a place。三焦具有疏通水道、运行水液的功能，故译为 drainage officer。

引例 Citations:

◎上焦如雾，中焦如沤，下焦如渎，故三焦者，犹之决渎之官，合中上而归于下，水道由之出焉。(《黄帝素问直解》)

（三焦的功能，上焦像雾一样，中焦像沤物池一样，下焦像水沟一样。所以，三焦就好像疏通水道的官员，合上焦、中焦的水液而汇集于下焦，水液排泄的通道由此而形成。）

The function of the upper energizer is like fog, the middle energizer a fermentor, and the lower energizer a drainer. Therefore, triple energizer is like a drainage officer, bringing the water in the upper and middle energizers to the lower energizer, thus forming the passage for water discharge. (*Direct Interpretation of Plain Conversation in Yellow Emperor's Internal Canon of Medicine*)

◎决，通也；渎，水道也。上焦不治，则水泛高原；中焦不治，则水留中脘；下焦不治，则水乱二便。三焦气治，则脉络通而水道利，故曰决渎之官。(《类经·藏象类》)

（决，疏通；渎，水道。上焦不能治理，则水湿泛滥于胸膈以上；中焦不能治理，则水湿停留中脘；下焦不能治理，则水湿导致二便失常。三焦之气正常，则脉络通畅而水道通利，所以称为决渎之官。）

Jue (决) means dredging and *du* (渎) means waterways. Water will attack the heart and the lung if the upper energizer fails to perform its functions; water retention will occur in the spleen and stomach if the middle energizer fails to play its role; urine and defecation disorders will arise if the lower energizer does not work properly. When the qi in triple energizer keeps harmony, the meridians will be unblocked and the flow of waterways will be smooth, hence the name "drainage officer" for triple energizer. (*Classified Classics*) yuánshén zhī fǔ

元神之府

House of Original Spirit

先天之神贮藏活动的地方。元神，即先天之神，为父母两精结合，随胚胎的形成发育而生之神。脑具有主宰生命活动、主意识思维和感觉运动的生理功能。脑藏元神，为元神的活动提供物质基础，故称脑为元神之府。张锡纯《医学衷中参西录·人身神明论》认为："脑中为元神，心中为识神。元神者，藏于脑，无思无虑，自然虚灵也；识神者，发于心，有思有虑，灵而不虚也。"人的思维、意识是精神活动的高级形式，以先天元神为基础，结合后天识神，在脑和心的共同调控下，对外界客观事物进行分析、谋虑、记忆，形成意识、思维、情志等精神活动。因此，元神对于生命活动极其重要，元神存则生命立，元神败则生命息。

The term refers to the place for accommodating original spirit. Original spirit, also known as inborn spirit, is what develops from the embryo as a result of sperm-egg binding. The brain is primarily involved in governing life activities, mental activities, senses, and movements. It stores original spirit and provides material basis for its activities. Hence the brain is called the house of original spirit. According to the section "Discussion on the Spirit of Human Body" of *Records of Chinese Medicine with Reference to Western Medicine* written by Zhang Xichun, "The brain houses original spirit; the heart governs conscious spirit that is acquired later. Original spirit in the brain is natural, void, and bright, free from meditation and deliberation, whereas conscious spirit in the heart involves meditation and deliberation, and is bright but not void." Higher levels of mental activities such as thinking, consciousness, and emotions are based on both original spirit and conscious spirit, and are jointly regulated by the brain and the heart through analyzing, planning, and memorizing objective things in the world. Therefore, original spirit is extremely important for life activities. Life exists with original spirit and ends without it.

【曾经译法】 supreme mental palace (brain); THE RESIDENCE OF MIND; the palace of the mind; the house of primordial mind; house of the original spirit; house of mental activity; brain

【现行译法】 house of mental activities; house of cerebral spirit; brain; house of mentality; seat of mental activity; fu-viscera of mental activity; house of (the) original spirit

【标准译法】 house of original spirit

【翻译说明】 元神，即先天之神，为父母两精结合。"元"有本原的意思，original 的意思是"原始的；最初的"，与"元"的意思相符。"神"按照约定俗成的术语翻译原则，译为 spirit。译词 residence 表示住所、住房，尤指宅第、豪宅；palace 指王宫、宫殿、总统府，尤指英国的王室，豪华住宅；seat 常指座位、席位。按照约定俗成的原则，选用 house (a building for people to live in, usually for one family)。

引例 Citations:

◎脑为元神之府，而鼻为命门之窍。(《本草纲目》卷三十四)
　　(脑是元神所在的地方，而鼻为命门的孔窍。)

The brain is where original spirit is housed, whereas the nose is the orifice of life gate. (*Compendium of Materia Medica*)

◎脑为元神之府，精髓之海，实记性所凭也。(《类证治裁》卷四)
　　(脑是元神所在的地方，精髓汇集之处，实际上记性依赖于脑。)

The brain is where original spirit stays and where essence converges. In fact, memory relies on the brain. (*Categorized Patterns with Clear-cut Treatments*)

◎夫脑为元神之府，清阳聚会之处。（《医法圆通》卷四）

（脑是元神所在的地方，人体清阳之气汇聚的场所。）

The brain is where original spirit stays and where lucid yang converges. (*Medical Law Tact*)

升降出入

Ascending, Descending, Exiting, and Entering

气运动的四种基本形式。升降，是气的上下运动；出入，是气的内外运动。气运动的形式多种多样，包括上升和下降、外出和内入、吸引和排斥、发散和凝聚等对立的形式。中医学着重论述了气的升降出入运动，认为"升降出入，无器不有"。人体之气运动的升与降、出与入是对立统一的矛盾运动，广泛存在于机体内部。一方面，升与降、出与入，以及升降与出入之间既相互制约，又相互促进，保持着协调状态。另一方面，虽然从某个脏腑的局部生理特点来看有所侧重，如肝、脾主升，肺、胃主降等，但从整个机体的生理活动来看，升与降、出与入之间必须协调平衡。只有这样，人体之气的运动才能正常，各脏腑的生理功能才能正常发挥。因此，气机升降出入的协调平衡是保证生命活动正常进行的重要环节。

The term refers to the four basic forms of qi movement. Ascending and descending are the upward and downward movement of qi, while exiting and entering are the outward and inward movement of qi. There is a variety of forms of qi movement, including the pair of opposites such as ascending and descending, exiting and entering, attracting and repelling, spreading and condensing. Traditional Chinese medicine focuses on the qi movement of ascending, descending, exiting, and entering, believing that "nothing can exist without qi movement." Ascending and descending as well as exiting and entering of qi are contradictory movements of the unity of opposites, which are extensively present in the human body. For one thing, ascending versus descending, exiting versus entering, as well as ascending and descending versus exiting and entering are mutually restrictive and mutually reinforcing, thus maintaining harmony. For another, although a certain form of qi movement has dominance over a certain organ, e.g., the liver and the spleen are primarily involved in ascending qi, while the lung and the stomach are primarily involved in descending qi, the balance between ascending and descending, exiting and entering must be coordinated from a holistic perspective of the human body. Only in this way can qi movement and visceral functions in the human body be normal. Therefore, a coordinated balance of qi movement, i.e., ascending and descending, exiting and entering, plays an important part in maintaining normal life activities.

【曾经译法】 ascending, descending, exiting, entering; ascending-descending and coming in-going out

【现行译法】 ascending, descending, out-going and in-going; ascending, descending, exiting, and entering; ascending, descending, going out and coming in; upward, downward, inward and outward movement

【标准译法】 ascending, descending, exiting, and entering

【翻译说明】 按照中医术语翻译简洁性、回译性和约定俗成原则，"升降出入"译为 ascending, descending, exiting, and entering。

引例 Citations:

◎出入废则神机化灭，升降息则气立孤危。故非出入，则无以生长壮老已；非升降，则无以生长化收藏。是以升降出入，无器不有。(《素问·六微旨大论》)

(凡动物类的呼吸停止，那么其生命也就会立即消灭；凡植物类的阴阳升降停止，那么其活力也就立即委顿。因此说没有出入，就不可能由生而长、而壮、而老、而死亡。没有升降，就不能由生而长、而开花、而结实、而收藏。所以气的升降出入运动，凡是有形之物都具有。)

When qi ceases exiting and entering, vital activities shall vanish; when qi ceases ascending and descending, qi configuration shall perish. Therefore, without exiting-entering of qi, there will be no birth, growth, maturity, senility, or death; without ascending-descending of qi, there will be no germination, growth, flowering, reaping, or storage. Consequently, ascending, descending, exiting, and entering of qi are found in every form of life. (*Plain Conversation*)

◎无升降则无以为出入，无出入则无以为升降，升降出入，互为其枢者也。（《读医随笔·升降出入论》）

（没有升降，也就没有了出入；没有出入，也就没有了升降。升降与出入之间，互为其发挥重要作用的部分。）

There is no exiting-entering of qi if there is no ascending-descending of qi, and vice versa. Ascending-descending and exiting-entering are important to each other. (*Random Notes While Reading About Medicine*)

津血同源

Body Fluids and Blood Are of the Same Origin.

津液和血都来源于水谷精气，二者相互滋生，相互转化，同出一源，相互影响的关系，称为津血同源。首先，津液和血同为液体，均属阴性，都来源于脾胃运化的水谷精微，皆具有滋润濡养作用，二者相互为用，共同完成滋养人体的作用。其次，二者在循行输布过程中可相互转化，津液从脉外注入脉内则成为血；血中的水液渗出脉外，则成为津液。正由于津液和血密切相关，所以在病机上也常相互影响，如失血过多，可导致津液的损伤，出现口渴、尿少、皮肤干燥等病理改变；反之，严重的伤津脱液，也会影响到血液，导致血脉空虚，津枯血燥等病变。

The term means that both body fluids and blood are derived from the essence of food and drinks. They are of the same source. They nourish, transform, and affect each other. First, both body fluids and blood are liquids, pertaining to yin. They originate from the essence of food and drinks, and are transported and transformed by the stomach and the spleen. They moisten and nourish each other, and jointly nourish the human body. Second, body fluids and blood can transform into each other in the course of circulation and distribution. Body fluids are transformed into blood when they enter the blood vessels; water in the blood seeps out of the vessels and is transformed into body fluids. It is precisely because of the close relationship between body fluids and blood that they affect each other in terms of pathogenesis. For example, excessive blood loss may damage body fluids, resulting in thirst, less urine, dry skin, and other pathological changes. Conversely, serious damage of body fluids will also affect the blood, causing blood deficiency, exhaustion of body fluids, and blood dryness, etc.

【曾经译法】 Body fluid and blood are derived from the same source; The body fluid and blood are of the same origin; Body fluid and the blood are derived from the same source; Liquid and blood are of the same source

【现行译法】 body fluid and blood derived from the same source; Body fluids and blood are derived from a common source; body fluid and blood sharing the same origin/source; body fluids and blood being of the same source; homogeny of clear fluid and blood; homogeny of fluid and blood; fluid and blood from same source

【标准译法】 Body fluids and blood are of the same origin.

【翻译说明】 "津血同源"强调"根源"，选用 origin。译词 homogeny 侧重有同样的形式、结构，不符合文意；share 可表达 same 之意。因此，译为 Body fluids and blood are of the same origin 在回译性层面更贴近源语。

引例 Citations:

◎中焦出气如露，上注溪谷，而渗孙脉，津液和调，变化而赤为血。(《灵枢·痈疽》)

(在中焦化为营气，像雾露一样，注入到组织间隙，渗入到孙络，与津液调和后，变成红色的血液。)

The nutrient-qi is transformed in the middle energizer. Like fog and dew, it enters the interstitial space, infuses into the minute collaterals, and blends in the body fluids before being transformed into blood. (*Spiritual Pivot*)

◎津液者，血之余，行乎脉外，流通一身，如天之清露。(《明医杂著·风症》)

(津液是血液溢出的部分，运行于脉外，流通于全身，好像自然界洁净的露水。)

Body fluids are the surplus of blood, which flow outside the blood vessels and circulate throughout the human body like clean dew in nature. (*Miscellaneous Writings of Famous Physicians of the Ming Dynasty*)

◎津亦水谷所化，其浊者为血，清者为津。以润脏腑、肌肉、脉络，使气血得以周行通利而不滞者此也。（《读医随笔·气血精神论》）

（津液也是由饮食水谷所化生，其中稠浊的部分为血液，清稀的部分为津液。以滋润脏腑、肌肉和脉络，使气血能够循行通畅而不涩滞的即是津液。）

Food and drinks can be transformed into body fluids, in which the thick part is blood and the thin part is fluid. The fluids are what moisten the zang-fu organs, muscles, and blood vessels so that qi and blood can flow smoothly without impediment. (*Random Notes While Reading About Medicine*) xuèhàn tóngyuán

血汗同源

Blood and Sweat Are of the Same Origin.

血汗同源是指血液和汗液共同来源于水谷精微，均依赖于津液所化的关系。中医认为血液的成分是营气和津液，其中血液渗出脉外者就形成津液。津液在阳气的蒸化作用下出于皮肤外则为汗液，所以有"血汗同源"之说。血汗同源提示我们，汗多不仅伤津液，也会伤血；失血者，不仅津液受伤，汗液亦无。因此，对于失血患者，临床上不宜用发汗等疗法，否则将重伤津液而加重病情；对于多汗津亏患者，也不宜用放血和破血方法，否则也将会再次损伤津血而加重病情。故张仲景《伤寒论》提出"衄家不可发汗""亡血家不可发汗"。

The term means that both blood and sweat originate from food and drinks and are dependent on the transformation of body fluids. According to traditional Chinese medicine, blood is composed of nutrient-qi and body fluids, in which the part that seeps out of the blood vessels is transformed into body fluids. Body fluids are turned into sweat when they evaporate to skin under the steaming function of yang-qi, hence the saying "blood and sweat are of the same origin." The saying suggests that excessive sweat damages not only body fluids but also blood; and the loss of blood damages not only body fluids but also sweat. Therefore, for hemorrhagic patients, sweating method should be avoided; otherwise, body fluids will be seriously damaged and the condition worsens. In cases of excessive sweating and fluid deficiency, bloodletting and removing blood stasis by drastic methods should be avoided; otherwise, body fluids and blood will be seriously damaged and the condition will worsen. Therefore, according to Zhang Zhongjing's *Treatise on Cold Damage*, "sweating therapy should be avoided in patients with nosebleeds" and "sweating therapy should be avoided in cases of blood exhaustion."

【曾经译法】 Blood and sweat are derived from the same source; Blood and sweat share the same source; Blood and sweat have the same source

【现行译法】Blood and sweat have one and the same source; Blood and sweat share the same source; Blood and sweat share the same origin; blood and sweat being of the same source

【标准译法】Blood and sweat are of the same origin.

【翻译说明】单词 origin 侧重指事物的起源或由来，也指人的出身；source 基本意思是河流或瀑布的源头，也可引申指某物，尤其是抽象事物（如兴趣、消息、情报）的根源或来源。相比较而言，origin 语义更广，多指起源、发端、出身，强调源头。故"同源"译为 same origin 较妥。

引例 Citations:

◎夺血者无汗，夺汗者无血。（《灵枢·营卫生会》）

（失血过多的人，其汗也少；出汗过多的人，其血也少。）

Little perspiration is seen in patients with excessive hemorrhage, and blood deficiency is found in patients with profuse sweating. (*Spiritual Pivot*)

◎血汗同源，不宜并逆。（《伤寒易简》）

（血与汗有相同的来源，不应同时耗伤。）

Blood and sweat are of the same origin and should not be damaged simultaneously. (*The Concise Book of Cold Damage*)

qì zhǔ xùzhī

气主煦之

Qi Warms the Body.

气具有产生热量、温暖人体的功能。气的温煦作用主要体现在以下几个方面：一是产生热量，维持体温的相对恒定。气是体内产热的物质基础，气在运动变化过程中不断产生热量，以温暖机体；此外，卫气控制汗孔的开合，通过调节汗液的排泄以调节体温的相对恒定。二是温煦脏腑、经络等组织器官，维持各自的生理功能。三是维持精、血和津液等液态物质的运行。气的温煦功能减退，产热过少，则可出现体温偏低，四肢不温，脏腑功能减退，精、血、津液运行迟滞不畅等病理表现。

Qi generates heat and warms the human body. Its warming function is mainly embodied in the following aspects. First, qi generates heat and maintains relatively constant body temperature. Qi is the material basis of heat production in the body. It continuously generates heat in its movement to warm the body. Besides, defense qi controls the opening and closing of sweat pores and regulates body temperature by regulating the excretion of sweat. Second, qi warms the zang-fu organs, meridians, and other tissues to ensure their physiological functions. Third, qi maintains the circulation of liquid substances such as essence, blood, and body fluids. Weakened warming function of qi and reduced heat production may cause such pathological changes as low body temperature, cold limbs, visceral dysfunction, and unsmooth circulation of essence, blood, and body fluids.

【曾经译法】Qi dominates warmth

【现行译法】warming function of qi; qi warming body; qi governing warmth

【标准译法】Qi warms the body.

【翻译说明】"气主煦之"为一个完整的句子，考虑简洁性原则，将其译为 Qi warms the body。

引例 Citations:

◎气主呴之，血主濡之。（《难经·二十二难》）

（气的功能是温煦人体，血的功能是滋养人体。）

Qi warms the human body, while blood nourishes and moistens it. (*Canon of Difficult Issues*)

◎气主呴之者，谓气煦嘘往来，熏蒸于皮肤分肉也。（《难经正义》）

（气主呴之，是说气温煦往来，熏蒸人体皮肤肌肉。）

Qi warming the body means qi produces heat to "steam" human skin and muscles. (*Differentiating the Meaning of "Canon of Difficult Issues"*)

◎气主煦之，百骸假是而温充。（《太医局诸科程文格》卷五）

（气的功能是温煦，人体全身通过气而得到温养。）

Qi warms the human body. Through qi the whole body is warmed and nourished. (*Tests of All Subjects by Imperial Medical Bureau*) xuè zhǔ rúzhī

血主濡之

Blood Nourishes and Moistens the Body.

血液具有营养和滋润人体的作用。血液由营气和津液所组成，营气乃水谷精微中之精纯部分所化生，津液可濡润全身，故血液的主要功能即是营养和滋润作用。血液行于脉中，循脉运行全身，内至五脏六腑，外达皮肉筋脉，对全身各脏腑组织不断地发挥着营养和滋润作用，以维持其正常的生理功能，保证人体生命活动的正常进行。若血液充足，营养滋润作用正常，则面色红润，视物清晰，肌肉丰满壮实，肌肤、毛发光泽，筋骨强劲，感觉灵敏，运动灵活。否则，血液亏虚，营养滋润功能减弱，可出现面色萎黄，视物昏花，唇甲色淡，皮毛枯槁，肌肉消瘦，筋骨痿软，肢体麻木，运动不灵活，脉细等症状。

Blood, composed of nutrient qi and body fluids, provides nutrients and moisture for the human body. Nutrient qi is the refined essence transformed from the essence of food and drinks; body fluids are to moisten the whole body. Therefore, the primary function of blood is nourishing and moistening. Blood circulates in the blood vessels throughout the body, reaching the zang-fu organs, skin, muscles, tendons, and vessels, constantly nourishing and moistening them to maintain their normal physiological functions and ensure life activities. Reddish complexion, clear vision, strong muscles, bones, and tendons, lustrous skin and hair, quick perception as well as flexibility in physical movement are evidences of blood sufficiency and the normal function of blood in nourishing and moistening. Otherwise, sallow complexion, blurred vision, pale lips and nails, dry hair and skin, muscle wasting, flaccidity of tendons and muscles, limb numbness, inflexibility in physical movement, and thready pulse may occur.

【曾经译法】Blood dominates nourishment; Blood dominates moisture and
　　　　　　nourishment

【现行译法】blood serving nutritive function; Blood is responsible for moistening and nourishment; blood being responsible for nurturing body; blood governing moisture and nourishment

【标准译法】Blood nourishes and moistens the body.

【翻译说明】单词 nourish 指给人、动物或植物提供食物以使其存活、生长，其名词形式是 nourishment；moisten 的意思是"湿润"（to moisten something means to make it slightly wet），其名词形式是 moisture；nurture 强调养育、滋长、助长。"血主濡之"指血液具有营养和滋润人体的作用，故译为 Blood nourishes and moistens the body 较妥。

引例 Citations:

◎气主呴之，血主濡之。（《难经·二十二难》）

（气的功能是温煦人体，血的功能是滋养人体。）

Qi warms the human body, while blood nourishes and moistens it. (*Canon of Difficult Issues*)

◎血主濡之者，谓血濡润筋骨，滑利关节，荣养脏腑也。（《难经正义》）

（血主濡之，是说血液能够滋润筋骨，使关节滑利，营养脏腑。）

Blood nourishing and moistening the human body means blood can moisten bones and tendons, lubricate joints, and nourish the zang-fu organs. (*Differentiating the Meaning of "Canon of Difficult Issues"*)

◎血主濡之，血虚则不能濡润筋络，故筋急也。（《注解伤寒论》卷一）

（血的功能是滋养，血虚不能滋养筋脉，所以导致筋脉挛急。）

Blood has the function of nourishing and moistening the human body. In cases of blood deficiency, spasm of tendons may occur due to the failure of blood to nourish them. (*Annotated "Treatise on Cold Damage"*)

气为血帅

Qi Is the Commander of Blood.

　　气对血而言，有化生、推动和统摄的作用，概称为"气为血帅"。一是气能生血，即气参与并促进血液的生成，气旺则血充，气虚则血少，气虚日久常可导致血液生成不足而见血虚证。二是气能行血，即气的推动作用是血液运行的动力，气行则血行，气止则血止，如果气虚推动无力，或气滞血行不利，可导致血行迟缓，甚至瘀血；若气机逆乱，升降出入失常，影响到血液的正常运行，血随气逆，或血随气陷，而见出血现象。三是气能摄血，即气具有统摄血液在脉管中运行，防止其逸出脉外的功能。若气虚固摄作用减弱，可导致尿血、便血、崩漏、紫癜等出血病症，称为气不摄血。

Qi can generate, promote, and control blood, which is generally described as "qi being the commander of blood." First, qi generates blood, i.e., qi is involved in and promotes the generation of blood. When qi is abundant, blood will be sufficient. When qi is weak, blood will be deficient. Prolonged qi deficiency often causes insufficient generation of blood and therefore blood-deficiency pattern occurs. Second, qi promotes blood circulation, i.e., qi is the driving force of blood circulation. As qi flows, blood follows. When qi stops, blood flow stops. If qi is weak or stagnates, unsmooth or sluggish flow of blood or even blood stasis may occur. If there is qi disorder with abnormal ascending, descending, exiting or entering, blood circulation will be affected, and bleeding may occur as a result of abnormal blood flow following the adverse flow of qi or the sinking of qi. Third, qi contains blood. Qi has the function of controlling blood to flow in the vessels and preventing it from escaping out of the vessels. In the case of qi deficiency with weakened controlling function, hemorrhagic diseases may occur such as hematuria, hemafecia, metrorrhagia, metrostaxis, and purpura, which is described as deficient qi failing to control blood.

【曾经译法】 vital energy as the commander of blood; "QI" (VITAL ENERGY) AS THE COMMANDER OF BLOOD; Qi is the commander of blood; Qi acts as the commander of Blood

【现行译法】 qi as the commander of blood; qi being (the) commander of blood; Qi is the commander of blood; qi commanding blood

【标准译法】 Qi is the commander of blood.

【翻译说明】 目前国内外对"气"的翻译比较统一，即将其音译为 qi。将 "气"意译为 vital energy 不能表达出"气"具有温煦、气化、固摄、防御等作用。因此，只有音译才能较好地保留"气"的多元内涵。采用 A is B 的形式翻译"气为血帅"更有助于体现中医的象思维。

引例 Citations:

◎气为血帅，故调经必先理气。(《女科辑要》卷上)

(气是血的统帅，因此，调理月经必须先调理气。)

Qi is the commander of blood; therefore, qi should be regulated before menstrual regulation. (*A Summary of Gynecology*)

◎血随气逆者，用缪氏气为血帅法，如苏子、郁金、桑叶、丹皮、降香、川贝之类也。(《临证指南医案》卷二)

(血随着气而上逆时，用缪氏气为血帅的治法，用药如苏子、郁金、桑叶、丹皮、降香、川贝之类。)

In the case of bleeding due to the adverse flow of qi, follow Master Miao's approach that qi is the commander of blood, using *suzi* (*Fructus Perillae*, perilla fruit), *yujin* (*Radix Curcumae*, curcuma root), *sangye* (*Folium Mori*, mulberry leaf), *danpi* (*Cortex Moutan Radicis*, moutan bark), *jiangxiang* (*Lignum*

Dalbergiae Odorifera, dalbergia wood), and *chuanbei* (*Bulbus Fritillariae Cirrhosae*, Sichuan fritillary bulb) to treat it. (*Case Records: A Guide to Clinical Practice*)

血为气母

Blood Is the Mother of Qi.

血对气而言，有生气和载气的作用，概称为"血为气母"。一是血能生气，即血液循环流布周身，能够不断地为气的生成和功能活动提供营养，以维持气的正常生理功能，故血充则气旺，血虚则气少。二是血能载气，即气依附于血中，依赖血之运载而布达全身。气属阳，主动；血属阴，主静。故气必须依附于有形之血，才能正常流通。否则，血不载气，则气将漂浮不定，无所依附而散越，如大出血的患者，往往气亦随之脱失，形成气随血脱的危症；或血行瘀阻不畅，而引起气机郁滞不通。

Blood can generate and carry qi, which is generally described as "blood being the mother of qi." First, blood generates qi. Blood circulates all over the body, continuously providing nutrition for the generation and functional activities of qi to maintain its normal physiological function. Therefore, qi is vigorous when blood is abundant and qi becomes weak when blood is deficient. Second, blood is the carrier of qi, a vehicle to bring qi to the whole body. Qi pertains to yang and is dynamic; blood pertains to yin and is static. Therefore, qi must depend on tangible blood for normal circulation. Otherwise, qi will float and scatter if blood fails to carry qi and qi has nothing to depend on. For example, in patients with massive hemorrhage, qi will collapse, resulting in a deadly disease known as qi desertion following blood loss; or qi stagnation may occur when there is obstruction in blood circulation.

【曾经译法】 blood as the mother of vital energy; BLOOD IS THE MOTHER OF QI (VITAL ENERGY); Blood is the mother of qi; blood being the mother of qi; Blood is the material foundation of Qi

【现行译法】 blood being (the) mother of qi; Blood is the mother of qi

【标准译法】 Blood is the mother of qi.

【翻译说明】目前国内外对"气"的翻译比较统一，即将其音译为 qi。将"气"意译为 vital energy 不能表达出"气"具有温煦、气化、固摄、防御等作用。因此，只有音译才能较好地保留"气"的多元内涵。采用 A is B 的形式翻译"血为气母"更有助于体现中医的象思维。

引例 Citations:

◎夫载气者血也，而运血者气也。(《血证论》)

　　(承载气的东西是血，而运送血的东西是气。)

Blood carries qi, and qi transports blood. (*Treatise on Blood Syndromes*)

◎血者气之守，气者血之卫，相偶而不相离者也。(《傅氏眼科审视瑶函》卷五)

　　(血是气的守护，气是血的护卫，二者相伴而不分离。)

Qi and blood guard each other, so they are inseparable. (*A Close Examination of the Precious Classic on Ophthalmology*)

神机气立

Vital Activity and Qi Configuration

神机是生命存在的根本，是主宰调控生命活动的机制；气立是生命得以维持的条件，是自然界的气化运动。二者作为两个相对独立的概念，又密切相关，共同揭示了生命体生化运动及其内外环境的整体联系。

神机相对于气立而言，主要指神对生命体内气化活动的调控与主宰，是生命存在的内在根据。它通过有组织、有目的的自我调控和运动，实现了人体内环境的稳态，同时在气立过程的协助下，维持着人体内外环境的协调。

气立主要指生命体与自然环境之间"气"的交流与转化，也可以说是生命体与外环境之间的物质、能量、信息的交换活动，是生命体赖以生存的条件，也是神机调控作用的表现。神机与气立相辅相成，共同维持着生命体的正常生命活动。

Vital activity is the foundation of life. It embodies the mechanism of governing and regulating life activities. Qi configuration, meaning qi movement in nature, is the condition on which life is sustained. These two concepts, though relatively independent, are closely related. They jointly reveal the overall connection between the generating and transforming activities of a living organism and its internal and external environment.

Vital activity, relative to qi configuration, mainly refers to the regulation and control of qi movement in the human body, and is the internal basis of life. By means of organized and purposeful self-regulation and movement, it ensures a steady state of the internal environment (homeostasis) and maintains the coordination of the internal and the external environments of a human body with the assistance of qi configuration.

Qi configuration mainly refers to the exchange and transformation of "qi" between the living organism and the natural environment, i.e., the exchange of substance, energy, and information. It is the condition on which the organism depends for survival and the manifestation of the regulation and control of vital activity. Vital activity and qi configuration complement each other to maintain the normal life activities of the living body.

【曾经译法】 vital activity; mysterious mechanism (神机)

【现行译法】 vital activity; mysterious mechanism; SPIRITUAL MECHANISM (神机); vital activity and qi configuration; shenji (magic mechanism) (神机); qili (origination of qi) (气立)

【标准译法】 vital activity and qi configuration

【翻译说明】 各中医学词典多将该术语分为"神机"和"气立"两个词条。"神机"分别有 vital activity, mysterious mechanism, spiritual mechanism 和 magic mechanism 四种译法。"神机"侧重指生命体内的自我调控和运动，并不强调特定机制，故 vital activity 较其他几个直译版本更符合术语含义。"气立"侧重指气的交流与转化活动，与 origination of qi 相比，翻译为 qi configuration 更加贴切，且该译法与 vital activity 结构对等，合并构成短语更加准确精炼。

引例 Citations:

◎根于中者，命曰神机，神去则机息；根于外者，命曰气立，气止则化绝。(《素问·五常政大论》)

（生物的生命根源于内的，叫做神机，如果神离去了，则生机也就停止。生命根源于外的，叫做气立，如果在外的六气变化歇止，那么生化也就断绝了。）

What originates from the interior of creatures is called vital activity. Generation and transformation will stop when the vitality is gone. What originates from the exterior of things is called qi configuration. Generation and transformation will cease if qi activity stops. (*Plain Conversation*)

◎出入废则神机化灭，升降息则气立孤危。(《素问·六微旨大论》)

　　(凡动物类的呼吸停止，那么其生命也就会立即消灭；凡植物类的阴阳升降停止，那么其活力也就立即委顿。)

When qi ceases exiting and entering, vital activities shall vanish; when qi ceases ascending and descending, qi configuration shall perish. (*Plain Conversation*)

◎凡物之动者，血气之属也，皆生气根于身之中，以神为生死之主，故曰神机……物之植者，草木金石之属也，皆生气根于形之外，以气为荣枯之主，故曰气立。(《类经·运气类》)

　　(凡动物，乃血气之类，其生命之气都根源于身形之内，以神为生死的主宰，所以叫做神机……凡植物，即草木金石之类，其生命之气都根源于形体之外，以气为荣枯的主宰，所以叫做气立。)

With blood and qi, animals have their vitality rooted in the interior of the body with spirit dominating the life, which is called vital activity... On the part of plants and minerals, their vitality is rooted in the exterior with qi dominating the growth, which is called qi configuration. (*Classified Classics*) jīngmài

经脉

Meridian; Normal Pulse

经脉是经络系统的主干，是气血运行和感应传导的主要通道。经脉包括十二经脉、奇经八脉和十二经别三类。十二经脉，又称十二正经，有一定的起止、循行部位和走向交接规律，与脏腑有直接的属络关系。奇经八脉与十二正经不同，与脏腑没有直接的属络关系，相互之间也无表里关系，具有统率、联络和调节十二经脉气血的作用。十二经别，是十二经脉的离合出入部分，具有加强十二经脉相表里的两条经脉的联系和补充十二正经的作用。由于经脉学说的重要源头为脉诊实践，故中医经典中"经脉"一词也常与"病脉"相对，指正常脉象。

The term *jingmai* (in most cases translated as meridian) refers to the trunk routes in the meridian system. Meridians are the main pathways for the flow of qi and blood as well as the conduction of sensations, and are classified into three categories: twelve (regular) meridians, eight extra meridians, and twelve divergent meridians. The twelve meridians, also called twelve principal meridians, are directly connected with the zang-fu organs. They begin, connect, and end at particular points, running along fixed routes in particular directions. The eight extra meridians, however, unlike the twelve principal meridians, do not pertain to any zang-fu organs, nor are they exterior-interiorly related. They have the effects of governing, coordinating, and regulating qi and blood in the twelve meridians. The twelve divergent meridians are the branches which derive from, enter, leave, and join the twelve principal meridians. They strengthen the connection between the exterior-interiorly paired meridians and supplement the twelve principal meridians. As pulse diagnosis constitutes a major part of the origins of meridian theory, *jingmai* may also be used in Chinese medical classics to refer to normal pulse manifestation, as opposed to *bingmai* (morbid pulse).

【曾经译法】 meridian and vessels; meridian; channels and vessels; meridians; channels; CHANNEL; jing-mai (the channels); channel vessel

【现行译法】 meridians; channel; main meridian; meridian

【标准译法】 ① meridian ② normal pulse

【翻译说明】 该术语主要有两种用词选择：meridian 和 channel，其中 meridian 为多个中医术语标准所采用，用于称谓中医的"经络"或者"经脉"。而 channel 含义宽泛，泛指所有的通道，包括中医的经脉概念。本书建议采用 meridian 来翻译"经脉"。此外，在某些语境下，经脉可指正常脉象，译为 normal pulse。

引例 Citations:

◎经脉者，所以行血气而营阴阳，濡筋骨，利关节者也。（《灵枢·本脏》）

（经脉是通行血气，运转阴阳，濡润筋骨，滑利关节的。）

Meridians are the pathways through which qi and blood flow as well as yin and yang aspects are transported to nourish the body, moisten tendons and bones, and lubricate joints. (*Spiritual Pivot*)

◎经脉十二者，伏行分肉之间，深而不见。（《灵枢·经脉》）

（十二经脉，隐伏在体内而行于分肉之间，位置深不能看到。）

The twelve meridians run deep in the muscular interstice and therefore are invisible. (*Spiritual Pivot*)

◎必先知经脉，然后知病脉。（《素问·三部九候论》）

（必先知道正常脉象，然后才能知道有病之脉。）

Only when one has fully understood the normal pulse can he/she know what a morbid pulse is. (*Plain Conversation*)

络脉

Collateral

络脉是人体内经脉的分支，纵横交错，网罗全身。从分支大小而论，有别络、孙络。别络又称"十五别络"，是较大的和主要的络脉，主要功能是加强相为表里的两条经脉在体表的联系；孙络是细小的络脉，属络脉的再分支，由线状延展扩大为面状弥散，进一步加强了各组织之间的联系和气血的渗灌。

从阴阳属性而论，有阴络、阳络。阴络，即下行、在体内、属脏的络脉；阳络，即上行、在体表、属腑的络脉。从气血而论，有气络、血络。气络，以气的运行为主；血络，以血的运行为主。从脏腑而论，根据络脉分布部位，有脏络、心络、肺络、脑络、胃络等不同名称。络脉的主要功能是渗灌气血，以发挥其营养滋润作用。

Collaterals are the branches of meridians, forming an intricate reticulated network throughout the body. They are further divided into divergent and tertiary collaterals according to sizes. Divergent collaterals, also called "fifteen divergent collaterals," are the larger and major collaterals, which can strengthen the connection between the exterior-interiorly paired meridians on the body surface. Tertiary collaterals are further divisions of these collaterals, extending from linear connection to surface diffusion, to further strengthen the connection at tissue level and promote the infusion of qi and blood.

From the perspective of yin-yang property, there are yin collaterals and yang collaterals. Yin collaterals run downward and are in the interior, connecting with the zang-organs. Yang collaterals go upward and are in the exterior, connecting with the fu-organs. From the perspective of qi and blood, there are qi collaterals and blood collaterals. Qi collaterals are featured by qi flow while blood collaterals by blood flow. From the perspective of zang-fu organs, different names are assigned to collaterals according to their locations. For example, there are zang collateral, heart collateral, lung collateral, brain collateral, stomach collateral, etc. Collaterals are primarily responsible for supplying tissues with qi and blood, bringing their nourishing and moistening effects into play.

【曾经译法】 collaterals and subcollaterals; collateral; collaterals; collateral vessel; luo-mai (the collateral channels); network vessel

【现行译法】 collaterals; network vessel; collateral (meridian); collateral

【标准译法】 collateral

【翻译说明】 多个中医术语标准采用 collateral 翻译"络脉",与"经脉"一词的译文 meridian 构成形式上的对等。与译文 collaterals and subcollaterals 相比,表达更简洁;与译文 network vessel 相比,表达更精准,且富有中医特色。

引例 Citations:

◎诸脉之浮而常见者,皆络脉也。(《灵枢·经脉》)
（诸脉在浅表而经常可以见到的,都是络脉。）

All vessels on the surface and visible to the eyes are collaterals. (*Spiritual Pivot*)

◎凡诊络脉,脉色青则寒且痛,赤则有热。(《灵枢·经脉》)
（凡察看络脉的病变,脉呈现青色,是寒邪凝滞并有疼痛;脉呈现赤色,是有热的病症。）

In terms of diagnosis of the collaterals, blueness of the vessels indicates cold stagnation with pain, while redness of the vessels indicates heat. (*Spiritual Pivot*)

◎酒入于胃，则络脉满而经脉虚。（《素问·厥论》）

（酒进入胃中，就使络脉中血液充满，经脉反而空虚。）

When wine is ingested into the stomach, the collaterals will be filled with blood. The meridians, however, will be empty. (*Plain Conversation*)

六淫

Six Excesses

六淫，是风、寒、暑、湿、燥、火六种外感病邪的统称。一般认为，六淫与六气有密切联系，六气是指风、寒、暑、湿、燥、火（热）六种正常的自然气候变化。正常的六气变化不会使人发病，而当自然界气候发生异常变化，出现太过或不及，或非其时而有其气，以及气候变化过于急骤，机体不能与之相适应时，就会导致疾病的发生，此时的六气便成为六淫。

六淫的实质，是以自然界风、寒、暑、湿、燥、火六种气候变化的不同特征，与人体疾病情况下的临床表现相类比，寻找二者之间的相似关系，所确立的病因模型。它是依据人体证候特点对多种实体病因的六种综合归纳，是以机体整体反应性为基准的关于外界病因的综合性功能模型。

Six excesses refer to the six exogenous pathogens including wind, cold, summer-heat, dampness, dryness, and fire. Generally, six excesses are closely related to six qi which refers to the normal climatic variations in nature (wind, cold, summer-heat, dampness, dryness, and fire/heat). Normal climatic changes are not pathogenic. Nevertheless, when they become unusual, i.e., excessive or deficient, unseasonable, or sudden and violent, to the extent that the human body cannot adapt to the changes, diseases would then arise. In such cases, six qi becomes six excesses.

Six excesses are virtually the etiological model established for determining the causes of diseases by drawing an analogy between the characteristics of the climatic variations in nature (wind, cold, summer-heat, dampness, dryness, and fire) and clinical manifestations in the human body. They are the synthesis and summary of six etiological factors in accordance with the patterns identified in human, a comprehensive functional model of exogenous pathogens based on overall physical responses to different causes to figure out responses for various situations.

【曾经译法】 six exopathogens; six exogenous pathogenic factors; six climatic evils; SIX CLIMATIC EXOPATHOGENS; six excesses

【现行译法】 six climate conditions in excess as pathogenic factors; six excesses; adverse environmental conditions of wind, cold, dryness, dampness, fire and summer-heat

【标准译法】 six excesses

【翻译说明】 该术语中"淫"字有多种译法且各有侧重，大体分为直译与意译两种方式。直译为 excesses 可揭示该术语的本质内涵，同时在保证术语中医特色的基础上，避免了其他译法不能完整传达术语内涵的问题。

引例 Citations:

◎六淫者，寒暑燥湿风热是也。(《三因极一病证方论》卷二)

（六淫，指寒、暑、燥、湿、风、热六种邪气。）

Six excesses refer to six kinds of pathogenic factors, namely, cold, summer-heat, dryness, dampness, wind, and fire. (*Discussion of Pathology Based on Triple Etiology Doctrine*)

◎三曰六淫之病，风寒暑湿燥火外邪所侵者是也。(《泰定养生主论》卷三)

（第三，六淫病症，指风、寒、暑、湿、燥、火外感邪气侵犯人体。）

Third, six excesses refer to the exogenous pathogens including wind, cold, summer-heat, dampness, dryness, and fire that may invade the human body and cause diseases. (*The Main Discussion on Health Preservation*)

◎外因六淫而得者，亦当先调气，后依所感六气治之。(《医门法律》卷三)

（由于外感六淫而患病者，也应该先调理气机，然后根据所感受的六淫邪气分别治疗。）

Those who are adversely affected by six excesses should first have their qi regulated and then be treated individually according to the identified pathogenic factor. (*Precepts for Physicians*) qīqíng

七情

Seven Emotions

　　七情，是指喜、怒、忧、思、悲、恐、惊七种情志活动，是人体对外界刺激所产生的不同反应，一般情况下不会导致或诱发疾病。只有强烈或持久的情志刺激，超过了人体的生理和心理适应能力，损伤脏腑精气，导致其功能失调；或人体正气虚弱，脏腑精气虚衰，对情志刺激的适应调节能力低下时，才会导致疾病的发生。七情常常两种或两种以上情志交织致病，多损伤人体五脏，使气机紊乱，而且多引起精神心理疾病，病情较为复杂。

The term refers to seven emotional activities: joy, anger, anxiety, over-thinking, sorrow, fear, and fright. They are the emotional responses to external stimuli. In most cases, they would not cause or trigger diseases. Only when they become excessive in intensity or duration, exceeding the psychological and physiological adaptability of a human being, would essential qi of the zang-fu organs be impaired and functional disorders arise. Diseases would occur when healthy qi is deficient, zang-fu organs' essential qi is consumed, and the human body adaptability to emotional stimuli is lowered. Usually two or more emotions are interlaced to cause diseases, harming the five zang-organs, disturbing qi movement, and leading to psychological conditions that are oftentimes complicated to treat.

【曾经译法】 seven modes of emotion; seven emotions; seven affects

【现行译法】 seven emotions; seven affects

【标准译法】 seven emotions

【翻译说明】 该术语中"情"字的译法主要为 emotions 和 affects。其中
　　　　　　 emotions 为中文术语含义"情志活动"的直译版本，affects

则为基于对该术语含义的理解进行的拓展翻译。比较两者，affects 含义宽泛，泛指影响，而 emotions 可精准地传达出"情"字在此处的中医内涵，因而更加符合原意。

引例 Citations:

◎七情者，喜怒忧思悲恐惊……七情，人之常性，动之则先自脏腑郁发，外形于肢体，为内所因。（《三因极一病证方论》卷二）

　　（七情，即喜、怒、忧、思、悲、恐、惊……七情是人的常性，其伤人先从脏腑郁滞而发，在外表现于形体，为内生之病因。）

Seven emotions refer to joy, anger, anxiety, over-thinking, sorrow, fear, and fright... As part of human characteristics, seven emotions are endogenous factors that may cause diseases. They would adversely affect people's health when they are restrained in zang-fu organs and manifest themselves in the exterior. (*Discussion of Pathology Based on Triple Etiology Doctrine*)

◎妇人之不孕，亦有因六淫、七情之邪，有伤冲任。（《妇人大全良方》卷九）

　　（妇女不孕，也有因为六淫、七情邪气，损伤冲任经脉的情况。）

Infertility in women may result from the impairment of thoroughfare vessel and conception vessel caused by six excesses and/or excess of seven emotions. (*Complete Effective Prescriptions for Women's Diseases*)

◎天有六邪，风寒暑湿燥火也；人有七情，喜怒忧思悲恐惊也。（《原机启微》卷上）

　　（自然界有六淫邪气，即风、寒、暑、湿、燥、火；人有七情内伤，即喜、怒、忧、思、悲、恐、惊。）

There are six excesses in nature, namely, wind, cold, summer-heat, dampness, dryness, and fire, while people may suffer internal impairment by seven emotions, namely, joy, anger, anxiety, over-thinking, sorrow, fear, and fright. (*Revealing the Mystery of the Origin of Eye Diseases*) zhèngqì

正气

Healthy Qi

人体精、气、血、津液等生命物质和脏腑经络等组织结构的正常功能活动，以及基于此而产生的各种维护健康的能力，包括自我调节能力、适应环境能力、抗病防病能力和康复自愈能力。正气的旺盛取决于以下基本条件：一是脏腑经络等组织器官结构的完好无损；二是精、气、血、津液等生命物质的充沛；三是各种功能活动正常及相互间的和谐有序。其中精、气、血、津液是脏腑经络等组织器官功能活动的物质基础，只有精、气、血、津液充足，脏腑经络等组织器官的功能方能正常和协调，人体的正气才能充盛。由于精、气、血、津液对于正气的盛衰常具有决定性作用，因此，人们往往以精、气、血、津液的多少作为判断正气盛衰的重要依据。

The term refers to the normal functional activities of life substances (essence, qi, blood, fluids, etc.) and structures (zang-fu organs, meridians, etc.) of the human body as well as the capability to maintain health including self-regulation, adaptation to the environment, disease resistance, prevention, self-healing, and recovery. The abundance of healthy qi depends on the following conditions: (1) intact structures of tissues, zang-fu organs, and meridians, etc.; (2) sufficient supply of life substances including essence, qi, blood, and fluids; (3) normal function and interaction of all life activities. Among them, essence, qi, blood, and fluids are the material basis of all functional activities, and their abundance ensures the normal function and coordination between tissues and organs as well as a prosperous healthy qi. As essence, qi, blood, and fluids are the decisive factors for the condition of healthy qi, their conditions are often viewed as important bases for determining the status of healthy qi.

【曾经译法】 healthy qi; vital qi; genuine qi; zheng qi (the primordial principle); right qi

【现行译法】vital-qi; right qi; healthy qi; normal qi; body resistance; genuine qi

【标准译法】healthy qi

【翻译说明】"正"字被译为 healthy, vital, genuine, right, normal 等。若直译为 genuine 或 right，可能会引起歧义；normal 含义不够准确。较为合理的译法为 healthy 或 vital。从"正气"一词的中医内涵角度考虑，healthy 传达出的含义更加全面且贴切，更能体现"正气"的本质特征及其对于机体生命活动的重要意义。

引例 Citations:

◎五疫之至……不相染者，正气存内，邪不可干。（《素问·刺法论》）

（五种疫病的发病……不相互传染，是因为正气充实于体内，邪气就不能侵犯。）

In terms of the five kinds of pestilence... if there is no infection when the five kinds of pestilence occur, it is because healthy qi is abundant in the body and pathogenic qi has no way to invade. (*Plain Conversation*)

◎三部脉均等，即正气已和，虽有余邪，何害之有？（《注解伤寒论》卷一）

（寸、关、尺三部脉象相等，说明正气已经调和，虽然还有未完全清除的余邪，又会有什么损害呢？）

The pulse manifestations are equal at *cun* (寸), *guan* (关), and *chi* (尺), the three sections over the radial artery, reflecting that healthy qi is in harmony. In such cases, although pathogenic factors are not eliminated, what damage will there be? (*Annotated "Treatise on Cold Damage"*)

◎由脏腑虚弱，风冷邪气乘之，邪气与正气相击，则腹痛也。（《诸病源候论》卷三十七）

（由于脏腑虚弱，风冷邪气侵犯人体，邪气与正气相互搏击，所以导致腹痛。）

Pathogenic wind and cold invade the body due to the weakness of zang-fu organs, causing the fight between healthy qi and pathogenic qi, resulting in abdominal pain. (*Treatise on the Origins and Manifestations of Various Diseases*) xiéqì

邪气

Pathogenic Qi

　　各种致病因素的统称，包括存在于外界环境之中和机体内部自身所产生的各种具有致病性的因素，如六淫、疫气、七情内伤、饮食失宜、劳逸失度、外伤、虫兽伤、寄生虫及水湿、痰饮、瘀血、结石等。邪气对机体的损害作用主要体现为：一是导致生理功能失常，造成机体阴阳失调，脏腑经络的功能紊乱，精气血津液的代谢及功能障碍等；二是造成脏腑组织的形质损害；三是改变个体的体质特征，进而影响其对疾病的易患倾向；四是导致机体抗病、自愈能力的下降。

The term refers to all kinds of pathogenic factors, including those in the external environment and those inside the body. Examples are six excesses, pestilential qi, excess of seven emotions, dietary irregularities, lack of exercises or excessive labor, trauma, insect bites or animal injuries, parasites, water dampness, phlegm retention, static blood, and stones. Pathogenic qi may bring the following harms to the human body: (1) physiological abnormalities leading to yin-yang imbalance, functional disorders of zang-fu organs and meridians, and metabolic and functional disorders of essence, qi, blood, fluids; (2) damaging the integrity of zang-fu organs and tissues; (3) changing an individual's constitution and altering the predisposition to disease; and (4) impairing the body's resistance to disease and the ability to heal on its own.

【曾经译法】pathogenic factors; evils; PATHOGENIC QI; xie (evil) qi; evil qi

【现行译法】pathogenic factors; evil qi; pathogenic factor; pathogen; the evil qi

【标准译法】pathogenic qi

【翻译说明】该术语中"邪"与"气"两字均有两种译法。其中，"邪"直译为 evil，意思为"邪恶的、罪恶的"；意译为 pathogenic。

"气"音译为 qi，意译为 factor，相对于正气，"邪气"译为
pathogenic qi。为准确传达该术语"致病因素"的中医内涵，
根据上下文，有时也采用 pathogenic factor 的译法。

引例 Citations:

◎皮毛先受邪气，邪气以从其合也。(《素问·咳论》)

（皮毛先感受邪气，邪气就会侵入相表里的肺脏。）

When pathogenic qi attacks the skin and hair, it enters the lung to which the
skin and hair pertain. (*Plain Conversation*)

◎夫病之一物，非人身素有也。或自外而入，或由内而生，皆邪气也。
(《儒门事亲》)

（疾病这一现象，不是人身平素所有。或者从外而侵入，或者由
内部而发生，都是邪气所致。）

The occurrence of disease is not inherent, but caused by pathogenic qi resulting
from either external invasion or internal transformation. (*Confucians' Duties to
Their Parents*)

◎脉来应时，为正气内固，虽外感邪气，但微自汗出而亦解尔。(《注解伤
寒论》卷一)

（脉象与四时相应，为正气充实于体内，虽然外感了邪气，但微
微自汗出，邪气也能解除。）

When pulse manifestation is found to correspond to the four seasons, it indicates
abundance of healthy qi in the body. Though invaded by pathogenic qi, one can
have pathogens relieved with slight spontaneous sweating. (*Annotated "Treatise
on Cold Damage"*)

nù zé qìshàng

怒则气上

Rage Drives Qi Upward.

暴怒则肝气上逆，或血随气逆，并走于上。肝为风木之脏，既藏有形之血，又疏无形之气，而怒为肝之志，若大怒不止，则肝气疏泄太过，导致肝气上逆，甚者血随气上逆，临床表现为头胀头痛，面红目赤，急躁易怒，甚则呕血，或卒然昏厥等。长期郁怒不解，又可使肝失疏泄，导致肝气郁结，出现胸胁、乳房、少腹胀痛，善太息等；若肝气乘脾，又可出现腹痛、腹泻等症。

Rage leads to the adverse flow of liver qi or blood, making qi and blood flow upward. Liver is the organ that pertains to wind and wood, which stores tangible blood and promotes the flow of intangible qi. Anger is the emotion associated with the liver. Persistent excessive anger can make liver qi disperse excessively, leading to the upward counterflow of liver qi or even blood. Clinical manifestations include distending headache, redness of face and eyes, vexation, irritability, and even hematemesis, or syncope. Long-term depression and anger may also bring the failure of the liver to disperse qi, causing liver-qi stagnation characterized by distending pain in the chest, hypochondria, breasts, and lower abdomen, as well as preference for deep sighing, etc. If liver qi subjugates the spleen, abdominal pain and diarrhea may occur.

【曾经译法】 Anger causes the Qi (vital energy) of the liver to go perversely upward; anger arousing ascent of qi; ANGER MAY LEAD TO THE ABNORMAL RISING OF VITAL ENERGY; Rage causes the qi (of the liver) to flow adversely upward; abnormal rising of vital energy due to anger; Anger may lead to the abnormal rising of vital energy; Rage causes adverse flow of Liver-Qi

【现行译法】 adverse flow of the liver-qi caused by rage; Rage drives qi upward; rage causing adverse flow of liver Qi to go adversely upward; rage causing qi to flow adversely upward; Anger causes qi to rise; rage causing qi rising; Rages drive qi upward

【标准译法】Rage drives qi upward.

【翻译说明】"怒则气上"主要表达气相对于正常情况下的反方向运行。单词 drive 较之于 cause 和 give rise to，主动意义更鲜明；upward 在保留了中医内涵的同时，表达更加简明清晰。

引例 Citations:

◎怒则气上……怒则气逆，甚则呕血及飧泄，故气上矣。（《素问·举痛论》）

（大怒则使气上逆……大怒则使气上逆，严重时可以引起呕血和飧泄，所以说"气上"。）

Rage drives qi upward… Excessive anger leads to the adverse flow of qi, or even hematemesis and *sunxie* (diarrhea with indigested food). Therefore, "qi flows upwards." (*Plain Conversation*)

◎大怒则形气绝，而血菀于上，使人薄厥。（《素问·生气通天论》）

（大怒会导致形与气隔绝，血淤积于头部，使人发生暴厥。）

Rage disturbs yang qi and drives qi and blood upward to stagnate in the head, eventually resulting in syncope. (*Plain Conversation*)

◎其心刚，刚则多怒，怒则气上逆，胸中蓄积，血气逆留。（《灵枢·五变》）

（这种人性气刚强，刚强就会多怒，怒就会使气上逆，使气积聚胸中，血气留滞不畅。）

Being fiery and forthright, these kinds of people tend to get angry easily. When they get angry, qi will flow adversely upward and accumulate in the chest, causing unsmooth flow of qi and blood. (*Spiritual Pivot*)

思则气结

Over-thinking Binds Qi.

思虑过度，可导致人体气机郁滞不畅。思为脾之志，过度思虑，以致脾胃气机郁滞，升降不及，运化失职，表现为纳差食少，腹胀，便溏等症；日久则致气血生化不足，可见头目眩晕，倦怠乏力，肌肉消瘦等。另外，思虑太过，亦可暗耗心血，使心神失养，而见心悸、失眠、多梦等症。

Over-thinking can cause unsmooth flow of qi. Thought or thinking is the emotion associated with the spleen. Over-thinking may result in qi stagnation in the spleen and the stomach, inadequate ascending and descending of qi, and the failure of transportation and transformation. Its manifestations include poor appetite, abdominal distension, and diarrhea. Over time, it will lead to insufficient production of qi and blood, manifested as dizziness, fatigue, muscle wasting, etc. In addition, over-thinking may consume heart blood, deprive the heart spirit of nourishment, and cause such symptoms as palpitations, insomnia, and dream-disturbed sleep.

【曾经译法】 Mental anxiety makes the Qi (vital energy) of the spleen depressed; worry causing stagnation of qi; ANXIETY MAY LEAD TO STAGNATION OF VITAL ENERGY; Anxiety makes the qi (of the spleen) depressed; Anxiety makes qi depressed; anxiety making qi depressed; Over-thinking may lead to the depression of vital energy; the depression of the vital energy caused by over-thinking; anxiety making Qi depressed; Anxiety makes Qi depressed; Anxiety Making Qi Stagnation

【现行译法】 anxiety making qi depressed; anxiety causing qi stagnation; Anxiety makes qi depressed; Thought causes qi to bind; pensiveness causing qi to stagnation; pensiveness generating qi stuckness

【标准译法】Over-thinking binds qi.

【翻译说明】此处的"思"指思虑过度，并非焦虑。因此，anxiety 含义传达不够准确，pensiveness 含义较窄，侧重指"陷入负面情绪的沉思"，故采用 over-thinking 较为贴切。"气结"的"结"选用常用译词 bind。

引例 Citations:

◎思则气结……思则心有所存，神有所归，正气留而不行，故气结矣。（《素问·举痛论》）

（思虑则使气郁结……思虑太过，就使人的心思经常留存于某一事物，精神也集中于一处，以致正气留结而不行，所以说"气结"。）

Over-thinking causes qi to bind… Excessive thinking leads to the concentration of mind and spirit on a particular issue so that healthy qi is retained and fails to circulate properly. Therefore, "qi binds." (*Plain Conversation*)

◎思则气结，结于心而伤于脾也。（《景岳全书》卷十九）

（思虑则使气郁结，郁结于心，而伤及于脾。）

Over-thinking causes qi to bind. Qi stagnates in the heart, and the spleen may be affected. (*Jingyue's Complete Works*) xǐ zé qìhuǎn

喜则气缓

Excessive Joy Slackens Qi.

过度喜乐，可导致心气涣散不收。喜为心之志，是一种良性的情志反应，喜悦适度，可使气血和调，营卫通利，心情平静舒畅，以缓和精神紧张。但大喜过度，又易引起心气涣散不收，重者心气暴脱或神不守舍，表现出心神不宁，注意力不集中，失眠，甚则喜笑不休，语无伦次，举止失常。如《灵枢·本神》说："喜乐者，神惮散而不藏。"

Excessive joy slackens heart qi. Joy is the emotion associated with the heart and is a type of beneficial emotional responses. Moderate joy can regulate the flow of qi and blood, make nutrient qi and defense qi unobstructed, and maintain ease of mind and a relaxed mood, relieving mental tension. However, excessive joy can easily slacken heart qi. In severe cases, collapse of heart qi, absent-mindedness, restlessness, inattention, insomnia, and even hysterical laughing, incoherent speech, and other abnormal behaviors may occur. As stated in the section "Basic State of Spirit" of *Spiritual Pivot*, "excessive joy and happiness cause heart qi to disperse and spirit is no longer stored."

【曾经译法】 joy inducing sluggishness of qi; Over joy may lead to the sluggishness of vital energy; EXCESSIVE JOY MAKES THE QI (OF THE HEART) SLUGGISH; An excess of joy may lead to the sluggishness of vital energy; Joy induces sluggishness of qi; joy inducing sluggishness of qi; excessive joy inducing relaxation of qi; Excessive Joy brings about descent of Qi.

【现行译法】 over joy relaxing qi; excessive joy inducing relaxation of qi; excessive joy relaxing Qi (of heart); Joy causes qi to slacken; over-joy causing qi to slacken; Over-joy leads to sluggishness of heart qi

【标准译法】Excessive joy slackens qi.

【翻译说明】不同译本之间的区别主要在于对"缓"的理解，该词主要译为 slacken, sluggishness 或 relaxation。其中 sluggishness 强调因缺乏能量而行动缓慢，relaxation 主要指放松，slacken 为及物动词，指"to make less active; slow up"（使放慢，减缓），是较为贴切的译词。

引例 Citations:

◎喜则气缓……喜则气和志达，营卫通利，故气缓矣。（《素问·举痛论》）

（大喜则使气涣散……正常的喜乐则使气和顺，志意畅达，营卫之气通利，而过喜则可使气涣散。）

Excessive joy slackens qi... Moderate joy and happiness lead to harmony of qi, ease of mind, and smooth flow of nutrient qi and defense qi. Over-joy, nevertheless, makes qi slacken and dissipate. (*Plain Conversation*)

◎喜则气缓，志气通畅和缓本无病。然过于喜则心神散荡而不藏，为笑不休，为气不收，甚则为狂。（《医碥》卷一）

（喜乐则使人气舒缓，志意与气通畅和缓而无病。但喜乐太过，则会使心神散乱而不能内守，出现喜笑不休，气不收敛，严重时导致狂证。）

Joy and happiness make qi and will harmonious and well-regulated so that disease will not arise. However, excessive joy will make heart qi dissipate and unable to maintain inside, causing hysterical laughing and failure of qi to astringe. In severe cases, manic symptoms may occur. (*Stepping Stones for Medicine*)

◎心藏神，其志喜，喜则气缓，而心虚神散，故宜食酸以收之。(《本草从新》)

（心主藏神，在志为喜。过喜则使心气涣散，而致心气虚，心神失守，因此宜食用酸味的东西以收敛心气。）

The heart stores spirit and corresponds to joy in emotion. Excessive joy makes heart qi slacken and dissipate so that heart-qi deficiency and loss of mind may occur. Sour foods are advised to take to astringe heart qi. (*Renewed Materia Medica*)

悲则气消

Excessive Sorrow Exhausts Qi.

过度悲伤，可导致肺气耗伤。悲为肺之志，过度的悲哀，易使正气消耗，尤其易致肺气耗伤，宣发肃降失常，临床可见气短懒言，声低息微，神疲乏力，意志消沉，易伤风感冒等。

Excessive sorrow consumes lung qi because sorrow is the emotion associated with the lung. Excessive sorrow dissipates healthy qi, especially lung qi, which causes its dysfunction of ascending, dispersing, purifying, and descending. Clinical manifestations include shortness of breath, no desire to speak, low voice and faint breathing, lassitude, lack of strength, low spirit, susceptibility to colds, etc.

【曾经译法】 excessive sorrow dissipating qi; Sorrow may lead to the consumption of vital energy; SORROW MAKES THE QI (OF THE LUNG) CONSUMED; Excessive sorrow leads to consumption of qi; Sadness may lead to the consumption of vital energy; excessive sorrow leading to consumption of qi; Excessive sadness leads to Qi consumption

【现行译法】 excessive sorrow resulting in consumption of qi; qi consumption due to grief; Sorrow makes the qi consumed; excessive sorrow leading to consumption of Qi; Sorrow causes qi to disperse; sorrow causing qi consumption; lung qi consumption due to over-grief

【标准译法】 Excessive sorrow exhausts qi.

【翻译说明】 "消"主要译为 consume 和 disperse。根据汉语释义，"消"指耗伤、消耗。为区别"耗"，此处将"消"译为 exhaust。

引例 Citations:

◎悲则气消……悲则心系急，肺布叶举，而上焦不通，荣卫不散，热气在中，故气消矣。（《素问·举痛论》）

> （悲哀则使气消损……过度悲哀，则使心系挛急，肺叶张大，上焦之气不得宣通，营卫之气不得布散，气郁化热，热气在内耗损正气，所以说"气消"。）

Sorrow may exhaust qi... Excessive sorrow may lead to the contraction of the heart and the expansion of the lung, causing the failure of the upper energizer to disperse qi and the failure of nutrient qi and defense qi to be distributed. Therefore, qi is restrained and transformed into heat and the heat-qi in the interior impairs healthy qi; hence "qi is exhausted." (*Plain Conversation*)

◎悲则气消，消则脉空虚。（《针灸甲乙经》卷六）

> （悲哀则使气消损，气消损则使脉道空虚。）

Excessive sorrow exhausts qi, which leads to empty pulse. (*The A-B Classic of Acupuncture and Moxibustion*)

◎悲则气消，心志摧抑沮丧，则气亦因之消索。（《医碥》卷一）

> （悲哀则使气消损，意志受到挫折压制而沮丧，就会使气也因此而消散。）

Excessive sorrow exhausts qi. If one's will and intents are suppressed by frustration, one will feel depressed and qi will also be dissipated. (*Stepping Stones for Medicine*)

恐则气下

Excessive Fear Drives Qi Downward.

过度恐惧，可导致肾气不固，气泄于下。恐为肾之志，卒受恐吓，或长期恐惧伤肾，气趋下行，封藏不固，导致精气下陷耗泄的病变，临床可见二便失禁，男子遗精，女子月经紊乱或白带增多；由于精气耗损，又可见腰膝酸软、两足萎软等症。

Excessive fear can lead to insecurity and sinking of kidney qi because fear is the emotion associated with the kidney. Being subject to sudden fright or persistent fear can impair the kidney, causing kidney qi to flow downward and become unconsolidated, and lead to the sinking and exhaustion of essential qi. Clinical manifestations include fecal and urinary incontinence, seminal emission, menstrual disorders, or increased leucorrhea. As a result of the loss of essential qi, soreness and weakness of the lower back and knee, weakness of both feet, and other symptoms may occur.

【曾经译法】Fear causes the Qi (vital energy) of the kidney to sink; fear causing descent of qi; TERROR MAY LEAD TO THE COLLAPSE OF VITAL ENERGY; Fear causes the qi (of the kidney) to sink; Fear causes descent of qi; Fright causes sinking of qi; Terror may lead to the abnormal falling of vital energy; Fear leads to sinking of Qi; Fear Causing Sinking of Kidney-qi

【现行译法】fright causing sinking of qi; Fear causes qi to sink; Terror may lead to the sinking of qi; fear causing qi sinking; Fear causes qi sinking

【标准译法】Excessive fear drives qi downward.

【翻译说明】"恐"主要翻译为 fear，fright 或 terror，其中 fright 主要指突然产生的恐惧，terror 主要指暴行引起的恐慌，二词均不太合适。"下"的翻译主要有四种：sink, descent, collapse 和 abnormal falling，其中 falling 主要指规模、数量或力量的减少，descent 主要指从高处到低处的下落，collapse 指垮掉、崩溃。对应"怒则气上"的英译结构，将"恐则气下"译为 Excessive fear drives qi downward。

引例 Citations:

◎恐则气下……恐则精却，却则上焦闭，闭则气还，还则下焦胀，故气下行矣。（《素问·举痛论》）

（恐惧则使气下陷……恐惧则使人肾的精气下却，不能上交于心肺，以致上焦之气闭塞，上焦不通，则气返还而滞于下，就会使下焦胀满，所以说"气下行"。）

Excessive fear drives qi downward... Excessive fear may lead to the sinking of essential qi, making the kidney unable to coordinate with the heart and the lung, causing qi obstruction of the upper energizer, and leading to the return of qi and distension of the lower energizer. Therefore, "qi is driven downward." (*Plain Conversation*)

◎恐惧不解则伤精，精伤则骨痿痿厥，精时自下。（《灵枢·本神》）

（过度恐惧而解除不了就会伤精，精伤就会发生骨节酸痛以及痿、厥等病，并常有遗精的症状。）

Excessive fear without relief will impair essence, and the impairment of essence will cause soreness and weakness of bones, flaccidity, and syncope, accompanied with habitual seminal emission in most cases. (*Spiritual Pivot*)

◎惊则气乱，恐则气下，必伤肝肾。(《景岳全书》卷十九)

（受惊则使气紊乱，恐惧则使气下陷，必然损伤肝肾。）

Excessive fright causes derangement of qi and excessive fear causes sinking of qi. The liver and the kidney will inevitably be impaired. (*Jingyue's Complete Works*) jīng zé qìluàn

惊则气乱

Excessive Fear Drives Qi Downward.

突然受惊，可导致心气紊乱，气血失调。惊为突然遇见异常之象，如目击异物，突受惊吓等出现的恐惧心理，犹如人对外界不良袭击的一种退却保护性的心理反应。突然受惊，可使气行紊乱，导致心神失常的病变。临床可见心悸不安，惊慌失措，目瞪口呆，失眠易惊，甚至见语无伦次，哭笑失常，狂言叫骂，躁动不安等精神错乱的现象。

Sudden fear or fright may cause disorder of heart qi, which then leads to disharmony between qi and blood. Fright is one's response to a sudden event, for example, witnessing something unusual or being startled suddenly. It is a protective psychological mechanism for human beings to deal with negative external stimuli. Fright can cause disorder of qi movement, leading to deranged qi flow and abnormal mental states. Clinical manifestations include palpitations, restlessness, panic, insomnia, and being easily startled. Some patients may even have manic symptoms such as incoherent speech, fanatic crying and laughing, manic raving, and agitation.

【曾经译法】 fright causing disturbances of qi; Terror may lead to disorder of vital energy; FRIGHT LEADS TO DISTURBANCE OF QI; Excessive fright leads to disturbance of Qi

【现行译法】 disturbance of the flow of qi caused by fright; fright disturbing qi; fright disrupting qi; fright causing disorder of qi; qi disorder due to terror

【标准译法】 Excessive fright deranges qi.

【翻译说明】 "惊"主要翻译为 fright 和 terror，其中 terror 主要指暴行引起的恐慌，而 fright 指突然受到的惊吓、产生的恐惧，因而适用于此术语语境。"乱"可译为 derange，强调失常、紊乱、错乱，较之于其他译词 disturb, disrupt 或 disorder，含义更加准确，符合术语内涵。

引例 Citations:

◎惊则气乱……惊则心无所倚，神无所归，虑无所定，故气乱矣。(《素问·举痛论》)

（受惊则使气紊乱……惊骇则使人心无所主持，神无所归宿，思虑无所决定，而心气动荡散乱，所以说"气乱"。）

Excessive fright causes derangement of qi... Sudden fear or fright leads to palpitations, mental distraction, and hesitation. Therefore, qi is deranged. (*Plain Conversation*)

◎惊泄者，因心受惊，惊则气乱，心气不通，水入谷道而泄。(《脉因证治》卷二)

（惊泄，是因为心受到惊吓，受惊则使气紊乱，心气不通畅，水液流入肠道而发生泄泻。）

Fright diarrhea occurs as the heart is startled. Fright causes derangement of qi, leading to the obstruction of heart qi and the inflow of water-fluid to intestines, which then causes diarrhea. (*Symptoms, Causes, Pulses, and Treatments*)

◎盖惊自外至者也，惊则气乱，故脉动而不宁。(《金匮要略广注》卷下)

（大概惊从外而来，受惊则使气紊乱，所以脉搏跳动而不安宁。）

Fright is derived from external stimuli. It may cause derangement of qi. Therefore, the patient's pulse feels restless. (*Extensive Annotations on "Essential Prescriptions of the Golden Cabinet"*) hán zé qìshōu

寒则气收

Excessive Cold Causes Qi to Contract.

寒邪侵袭人体，可使气机收敛，腠理、经络、筋脉收缩而挛急。寒邪致病具有收缩牵引之性，寒邪侵及肌表，则毛窍腠理闭塞，卫阳被郁不得宣泄，可见恶寒、发热、无汗等症状；寒邪侵及血脉，则气血凝滞，血脉挛缩，可见头身疼痛，脉紧；寒邪伤于经络关节，则经脉收缩拘急，可见关节屈伸不利、或冷厥不仁等症状。

Pathogenic cold invades the body and causes qi to contract, leading to the contraction and spasm of interstices, meridians, tendons, and vessels. Cold-induced diseases are characterized by contraction. When pathogenic cold invades the surface of the skin and muscles, it closes the pores and muscular interstices, thus constraining the defensive yang from dispersion. Clinical manifestations include aversion to cold, fever, and absence of sweat. When cold invades the blood vessels, stagnation of qi and blood and spasm of blood vessels may occur, which may be manifested as headache and pain in the body with tight pulse. When cold invades meridians and joints, contraction and spasm of joints may arise, which can be manifested as inhibited bending and stretching or having cold and numb joints.

【曾经译法】 Cold induces contraction; Cold-evil renders the energy sluggish; COLD CAUSES CONTRACTION

【现行译法】 Cold renders yang-qi sluggish; Cold makes qi compact; cold astringing qi; cold contracting qi; cold causing qi to contract

【标准译法】 Excessive cold causes qi to contract.

【翻译说明】 以往各个翻译版本均以直译为主。其中"寒"均统一译为cold。"收"主要译为contract，sluggish，compact或astringe，其中contract更接近原文的"收缩、收敛"之意，因此选用。

引例 Citations:

◎寒则气收……寒则腠理闭，气不行，故气收矣。(《素问·举痛论》)

　　(遇寒则使气收敛……寒冷使人腠理闭塞，营卫之气难以运行，所以说'气收'。)

Excessive cold causes qi to contract... Excessive cold leads to closure of muscular interstices and obstruction of qi flow. Therefore, "qi contracts." (*Plain Conversation*)

◎寒则气收者，盖以身寒则腠理闭，卫气不得行于外，故脏腑之气收敛于内也。(《黄帝内经素问注证发微》卷五)

　　(寒则气收者，大概因为身体感受寒邪则腠理闭塞，卫气不能循行于体表，因此脏腑之气收敛于体内。)

The pathogenesis that excessive cold causes qi to contract is perhaps as follows: when human body is affected by pathogenetic cold, muscular interstices would be closed, and then defense qi would fail to reach the superficial part of the body. As a result, the qi of the zang-fu organs would be astringed inside. (*Annotations and Commentary* of *Plain Conversation in Yellow Emperor's Internal Canon of Medicine*)

◎寒则气收，宜辛散之，甘缓之。(《玉机微义》卷十六)

　　(寒邪则使气收敛，治疗宜用辛味药发散它，用甘味药舒缓它。)

Excessive cold causes qi to contract. Its treatment requires the use of pungent herbals to disperse qi and sweet medicines to relieve it. (*Detailed Explanation of the Jade Pivot*) jiǒng zé qìxiè

炅则气泄

Excessive Heat Causes Discharge of Qi.

暑热之邪致病，可使腠理开张，正气外泄。暑热之邪有升散之性，侵犯人体后可使人体腠理开张，迫津外泄，由于津能载气，故在津液外泄的同时，气无所依附也随津外泄，故临床除见口渴喜饮、尿赤短少等津伤之症外，往往可见气短、乏力，甚则气津耗伤太过，清窍失养而突然昏倒、不省人事。

Pathogenic summer-heat could give rise to the opening of muscular interstices and the discharge of healthy qi. Characterized by ascent and dispersion, pathogenic summer-heat forces fluids to discharge from open pores. Along with the loss of fluids, qi is also discharged as fluids carry qi. Clinically, it can be manifested as fluid consumption and qi deficiency. The former includes thirst with a desire for drinks and scanty dark-colored urine, while the latter includes shortness of breath and fatigue. When qi and fluids are exhausted in severe cases, sudden fainting and unconsciousness may occur due to the lack of nourishment in clear orifices.

【曾经译法】 fever leading to consumption of vital energy; heat leads to discharge of qi

【现行译法】 HEAT CONSUMES VITAL ENERGY; Heat leads to discharge of qi; Heat makes qi dispersed; fever resulting in dissipation of the yang principle; overheat causing qi leakage

【标准译法】 Excessive heat causes discharge of qi.

【翻译说明】 过热导致正气外泄。"过热"对应 excessive heat。"泄"的译法有 consumption（消耗），discharge（排放，流出），disperse（分散），dissipation（消散；浪费），leakage（泄露）等。基于该术语的中文释义，此处用 discharge 较为合适。

引例 Citations:

◎炅则气泄……炅则腠理开，荣卫通，汗大泄，故气泄。(《素问·举痛论》)

(遇热则使气外泄……暑热则使人的腠理开发，营卫之气运行通利，大汗出，气随汗液外泄，所以说"气泄"。)

Excessive heat causes discharge of qi... Excessive summer-heat makes muscular interstices open, brings smooth flow of nutrient qi and defense qi, and induces profuse sweating. Qi will leak out along with perspiration; hence "qi leaks." (*Plain Conversation*)

◎炅则气泄。今暑邪干卫，故身热自汗，以黄芪甘温补之为君。(《脾胃论》卷中)

(遇热则使气外泄。现暑邪侵犯于卫分，所以身体发热，自汗出，用黄芪甘温补气作为君药。)

Excessive heat causes qi leaking. Now pathogenic summer-heat invades defense qi, and fever and spontaneous sweat can be present. Sweet-warm *huangqi* (*Radix Astragali*, astragalus root), which supplements qi, should be used as monarch medicinal. (*Treatise on the Spleen and Stomach*) láo zé qìhào

劳则气耗

Overexertion Consumes Qi.

过度劳伤，常导致人体正气耗伤。过度劳作，常见呼吸喘息，汗出过多。喘息不止，使肺气内耗；汗出过多，则气随津泄，最终导致人体正气亏虚，尤其是耗伤脾肺之气，临床常见少气懒言、神疲乏力、四肢倦怠等症状。

Overexertion usually causes consumption of healthy qi. Overexertion leads to excessive panting and sweating. Excessive panting consumes lung qi, while over-sweating may lead to deficiency of healthy qi as qi could be discharged along with the loss of fluids. Consumption of healthy qi, especially lung qi and spleen qi, is thus developed. Clinically, it is often manifested as shortness of breath, no desire to speak, lassitude, lack of strength, and fatigue in the extremities.

【曾经译法】 overexertion may lead to consumption of vital energy; overexertion leading to consumption of qi

【现行译法】 OVER-EXERTION LEADING TO QI EXHAUSTION; strain makes qi consumed; overstrain leading to consumption of qi; overexertion leading to qi consumption; overexertion causing loss of qi; qi exhaustion due to extreme tiredness

【标准译法】 Overexertion consumes qi.

【翻译说明】 "劳则气耗"指过度劳伤导致人体正气损耗。"劳"的译法，更为普遍的说法是 overexertion。此处的"耗"指"损耗"，而非"枯竭"或者其他说法，故采用 consume。

引例 Citations:

◎劳则气耗……劳则喘息汗出，外内皆越，故气耗矣。(《素问·举痛论》)

（过劳则使气耗散……劳役过度，就出现喘息和汗出，使人体内外的正气皆泄越而耗散，所以说"气耗"。）

Overexertion consumes qi... It leads to panting, sweating, and leakage of healthy qi in the interior and exterior of the human body. Therefore, "qi is consumed." (*Plain Conversation*)

◎劳则气耗者，正以人有劳役则气动而喘息，其汗必出于外，夫喘则内气越，汗出则气外越，故气以之而耗散也。(《黄帝内经素问注证发微》卷五)

（劳则气耗者，正是由于人有劳役过度，就会扰动气机而出现喘息，汗液必然外出。喘息则使体内之气散越，汗出则使气向外散越，所以气因此而耗散。）

The reason why overexertion causes consumption of qi is that overexertion will disturb qi movement and lead to panting and sweating. Panting causes qi in the interior to disperse, while sweating causes qi to disperse outside. As a result, qi is consumed and dissipated. (*Annotations and Commentary* of *Plain Conversation in Yellow Emperor's Internal Canon of Medicine*)

◎盖劳则气耗而肺伤，肺伤则声哑。(《石山医案》卷下)

（大概过劳则使人气耗而肺受到损伤，肺损伤则使人声音嘶哑。）

Perhaps overexertion causes consumption of qi and lung qi is then impaired, which leads to hoarseness. (*Shishan's Case Records*)

邪正盛衰

Exuberance and Debilitation of Pathogenic Qi and Healthy Qi

邪正盛衰是指在疾病过程中，机体的抗病能力与致病邪气之间相互斗争所发生的盛衰变化。邪气侵犯人体后，一方面邪气对机体的正气有着损害作用，另一方面正气也对邪气产生抗御和驱除作用。邪正双方不断斗争的态势和结果，不仅关系着疾病的发生，而且直接影响着疾病的发展和转归，同时也决定病证的虚实变化。正邪相争，若正盛邪实，邪正斗争剧烈，多表现为实证；正气不足，邪气也不甚，则多表现为虚证；邪盛正虚，多形成较为复杂的虚实错杂之证。

The term refers to the change in strength (i.e., exuberance and debilitation) of healthy qi and pathogenic qi in their combat as diseases develop. Healthy qi may be impaired when pathogenic qi invades the body, but on the other hand, healthy qi can defend and expel pathogens. The tendency and the result of the combat will not only determine the occurrence of diseases, but affect the development, prognosis, and excess/deficiency of the condition. In the combat, if both healthy qi and pathogenic qi are exuberant, the fight will be fierce, and excess patterns may occur in most cases; if both healthy qi and pathogenic qi are debilitated, deficiency patterns may arise in most cases; if pathogenic qi is exuberant and healthy qi is debilitated, deficiency-excess complex patterns may be found in most cases.

【曾经译法】 prosperity and decline of the evil and the genuine; excess and weakness of Evil and vital Qi; EXUBERANCE AND DEBILITATION

【现行译法】 exuberance and decline of pathogenic factors and healthy qi; preponderance and decline; excess and decline; exuberance and debilitation

【标准译法】 exuberance and debilitation of pathogenic qi and healthy qi

【翻译说明】该术语的翻译主要在于"盛"与"衰"两个词的翻译。"盛"的选词有 exuberance, excess 和 preponderance;"衰"的选词有 decline 和 debilitation。大多数版本选用 exuberance 翻译"盛"字。而"衰"的翻译,本书建议使用 debilitation,因为 debilitation(衰弱)常用于医疗语境,指人由于疾病而变得虚弱无力。

引例 Citations:

◎实中有积,大毒之剂治之尚不可过,况虚而有积者乎?此治积之一端也,邪正盛衰,固宜详审。(《景岳全书·杂证谟》)

（病证实中有积聚,用药性峻猛的方药治疗尚且不能过量,况且正虚而有积聚的呢?这是治疗积聚的一方面,邪正的盛衰,因此应详细审察。)

Even when there are accumulations in the excess pattern, drastic medicinals cannot be overused, not to mention when there are accumulations in the deficiency pattern. This is one consideration in the treatment of accumulation. The exuberance and debilitation of healthy qi and pathogenic qi should be evaluated meticulously. (*Jingyue's Complete Works*)

◎须审生克顺逆之理,邪正盛衰之脉而治之。(《伤寒集验》卷一)

（必须审察五行相生相克顺逆的道理,邪正盛衰的脉象变化而进行治疗。)

Generation, restriction, over-restriction, and counter-restriction among the five elements and pulse manifestation in terms of exuberance and debilitation of pathogenic qi and healthy qi should be evaluated before treatment. (*Collection of Experience on Cold Damage*)

◎设不知岁气变迁，而妄呼寒热，则邪正盛衰无所辨。（《成方切用·方剂总义》）

（假若不了解岁运之气的变化，而不确切地称为寒热，那么邪正的盛衰就无从辨别。）

If one fails to understand the changes in dominant qi of the year, and only considers whether it is cold or heat, one cannot differentiate exuberance and debilitation of pathogenic qi and healthy qi. (*Effective Use of Established Formulas*)

真实假虚

True Excess with Pseudo-deficiency

病证的本质为"实"，但表现出"虚"的临床假象。一般是由于邪气亢盛，结聚体内，阻滞经络，气血不能外达所致，又称为"大实有羸状"。如热结胃肠的里热炽盛证，一方面有大便秘结、腹痛硬满、谵语等实热症状，同时因阳气被郁，不能四布，而见面色苍白、四肢逆冷、精神委顿等状似虚寒的假象。

The term refers to the clinical situation where the nature of a disease is excess, but instead, deficiency is manifested in disguise. It is caused by internal accumulation of hyperactive pathogenic qi obstructing meridians and restraining qi and blood from reaching outside. The pattern is also known as the "occurrence of deficiency manifestations in extreme excess." For example, when heat binds in the stomach and the intestines as in the pattern of intense interior heat, excess heat symptoms can be manifested as constipation, abdominal pain with rigidity and fullness, or even delirium. On the other hand, as yang qi is blocked inside and unable to disperse, pseudo-deficiency cold symptoms may occur such as pale complexion, reversal cold of the extremities, and lassitude.

【曾经译法】 asthenia-syndrome in appearance but sthenia-syndrome in nature; excess syndrome with pseudo-deficiency; REAL EXCESS WITH PSEUDO-DEFICIENCY

【现行译法】 syndrome of excess type with pseudo-deficiency symptoms; sthenia syndrome with pseudo-asthenia symptoms; true sthenia and false asthenia syndrome; true excess and false deficiency syndrome; excess syndrome with pseudo-deficiency symptoms; true excess with false deficiency; excess syndrome with pseudo-deficiency

【标准译法】 true excess with pseudo-deficiency

【翻译说明】各个翻译版本的不同之处在"真""实""假""虚"四个字上都有所体现。就"真假"而言，一般用的是 true 和 false 或前缀 pseudo-，其中前缀 pseudo- 常用于构成形容词和名词，表示"假的；伪的；冒牌的"；就"虚实"而言，excess 和 deficiency 已经成为"实"和"虚"约定俗成的译法。从"真实假虚"术语结构上看，此处应该是强调前者"真实"，因此用 with 连接，表示后者为伴随状态。

引例 Citations:

◎真实假虚之候，非曰必无，如寒邪内伤，或食停气滞，而心腹急痛，以致脉道沉伏，或促或结一证，此以邪闭经络而然，脉虽若虚，而必有痛胀等证可据者，是诚假虚之脉，本非虚也。(《景岳全书·脉神章》)

（真实假虚的现象，不是说必然没有，例如寒邪内伤，或者食积气滞，而出现心腹急痛，导致脉象沉伏，或促或结的病证，这是由于邪气闭阻经络而导致，脉象虽然像虚证，但必然有疼痛、胀满等症状可作为证据，这实为假虚的脉象，本质不是虚证。)

One cannot be so sure that the pattern of true excess with pseudo-deficiency manifestations does not exist. For instance, endogenous pathogenetic cold or food accumulation causes qi stagnation and may lead to acute pain in the heart and the abdomen with deep, hidden, abrupt or knotted pulse. It is caused by pathogenic qi blocking meridians. Although pulse manifestations may indicate deficiency, there must be such excess symptoms as pain and distension. This is the pulse manifestation of pseudo-deficiency, but not deficiency pattern in nature. (*Jingyue's Complete Works*)

◎虽真实假虚，非曰必无，但轻者可从证，重者必从脉，方为切当。(《脉义简摩》卷二)

（虽然真实假虚的现象，不是说必然没有，但病情轻的可以根据症状来治疗，病情重的必须根据脉象来治疗，才是正确的治法。）

One cannot be so sure that the pattern of true excess with pseudo-deficiency manifestations does not exist. While mild diseases should be treated in accordance with symptoms, serious diseases must be treated in accordance with pulse manifestation. This is the appropriate method. (*Interpretation on Pulses*) zhēnxū jiǎshí

真虚假实

True Deficiency with Pseudo-excess

病证的本质为"虚"，但表现出"实"的临床假象。一般是由于正气虚弱，脏腑经络之气不足，推动、激发功能减退所致，又称为"至虚有盛候"。如脾气虚弱，运化无力，可见脘腹胀满、疼痛（但时作时减）等假实征象。老年或大病久病，因气虚推动无力而出现的便秘也属此类。

The term refers to the clinical condition of a patient whose disease is deficiency in nature, but instead, excess is manifested in disguise. The phenomenon is mainly attributable to the deficiency of healthy qi in the zang-fu organs and meridians, leading to a decline in its propelling and stimulating functions. The term is also known as the "occurrence of excess manifestations in extreme deficiency." For example, deficiency of spleen qi, causing dysfunction of transportation and transformation, may result in such pseudo-excess symptoms as gastric and abdominal distension and pain (usually intermittent). Another case in point is constipation that occurs after a prolonged or serious illness or in aged patients due to inability of deficient qi to propel bowel movement.

【曾经译法】 false sthenia-syndrome in appearance but real asthenia-syndrome in nature; REAL DEFICIENCY AND PSEUDO-EXCESS; sthenia-syndrome in appearance and asthenia-syndrome in nature; true deficiency with false excess; deficiency syndrome with pseudo-excess symptoms; real Deficiency with pseudo-Excess

【现行译法】 deficiency syndrome with pseudo-excess symptoms; asthenia syndrome with pseudo-sthenia symptoms; true asthenia and false sthenia; true deficiency and false excess syndrome; true deficiency with false excess

【标准译法】 true deficiency with pseudo-excess

【翻译说明】 "真"指真实的病证本质，与临床假象相对，因此用 true

比较符合原意。"假"指假象，与真实的本质相对，译为
pseudo 比较符合原意。中医语境中的"虚"和"实"通常译
为 deficiency 和 excess。从"真虚假实"术语结构上看，此
处应该是强调前者"真虚"，因此用 with 连接，表示后者为
伴随状态。

引例 Citations:

◎况且世人之躯多真虚假实，本科之症多上热下寒。(《目经大成》卷一)
　　(况且普通人的身体多有真虚假实之证，眼科的病症多有上热下
　　寒之证。)

Moreover, average people are often found to have true deficiency pattern
with pseudo-excess symptoms, and their eye diseases often fall into the
pattern of upper heat and lower cold. (*The Great Compendium of Classics on
Ophthalmology*)

◎然至虚有盛候，则有假实矣；大实有羸状，则有假虚矣。(《医术》卷一)
　　(但极虚而呈现亢盛的征候，就有假实之象；大实而呈现虚弱的
　　状态，就有假虚之象。)

However, there may be excess manifestations when a deficiency pattern
develops to an extreme, and thus pseudo-excess symptoms occur; there may be
deficiency manifestations when an excess pattern develops to an extreme, and
thus pseudo-deficiency symptoms occur. (*Medical Art*)

阴阳失调

Yin-yang Disharmony

阴阳失调即阴阳之间失去平衡协调的简称。是指在疾病的发生发展过程中，由于各种致病因素的影响，导致机体阴阳双方失去相对的平衡与协调，从而出现阴阳偏盛或偏衰、阴阳互损、阴阳格拒、阴阳亡失等一系列病理变化。阴阳失调主要体现为寒、热性证候的变化。另外，中医学认为，各种致病因素作用于人体，都必须通过机体内部的阴阳失调才能形成疾病，所以，阴阳失调也是对人体各种功能性和器质性病变的高度概括。

The term is a brief way to refer to the loss of balance between yin and yang. Specifically, it denotes that during the development and progression of a disease, the relative balance and coordination between yin and yang is disrupted due to various pathogenic factors, which results in a series of pathological changes including relative exuberance or debilitation, mutual impairment, mutual repelling, and collapse of yin and yang. The breakdown of balance between yin and yang primarily manifests itself as cold or heat patterns. In addition, traditional Chinese medicine believes that pathogenic qi will not cause illnesses until the yin-yang balance of the human body is broken. Therefore, in this sense, the term is also a general statement denoting various functional and organic disorders.

【曾经译法】 IMBALANCE OF YIN AND YANG; incoordination between yin and yang; yin-yang disharmony; imbalance of yin and yang; disharmony of yin and yang; imbalance of Yin and Yang; incoordination of Yin and Yang; imbalance/disorder of yin and yang

【现行译法】 imbalance of yin and yang; imbalance between yin and yang; disharmony between yin and yang; yin-yang disharmony; breakdown of balance between yin and yang

【标准译法】yin-yang disharmony

【翻译说明】"失调"被译为 imbalance, incoordination, disharmony, disorder 或 breakdown of balance。其中，imbalance 侧重指对应事物比例或关系失调；incoordination 多指动作不协调；disharmony 强调整体不和谐；disorder 指整体局面混乱；breakdown 通常指系统故障或亲密关系破裂。世界中医药学会联合会标准等均采用 yin-yang disharmony 的译法。

引例 Citations:

◎人身所生疾病，未有不因阴阳失调，水火偏胜。(《冯氏锦囊秘录》卷十一)

（人体所发生的疾病，没有不是因为阴阳失调、水火偏胜而形成的。）

All human diseases are caused by yin-yang disharmony or the relative predominance of water or fire. (*Feng's Secret Records in Brocade Bag*)

◎夫诸虚百损，皆由阴阳失调，水火偏胜而来。(《家藏蒙筌》卷一)

（各种虚损性疾病，都是由于阴阳失调、水火偏胜而导致。）

All deficiency and impairment diseases are attributable to yin-yang disharmony or the relative predominance of water or fire. (*Comprehensive Secret Medical References of the Family*) yīnshèng zé hán

阴胜则寒

Yin Predominance Causes Cold.

机体在疾病过程中所出现的一种阴气病理性偏盛，功能抑制，热量耗伤过多，病理性代谢产物积聚的病理状态。阴气具有凉润、抑制、宁静等作用，阴气的病理性亢盛以寒、静、湿为特点，形成阴盛而阳未虚的实寒证，临床表现为形寒、肢冷、蜷卧、舌淡而润、脉迟等。导致阴胜则寒的主要原因多是感受寒湿阴邪，或过食生冷、寒邪中阻等，机体阳气难以与之抗争而致阴气病理性亢盛。

The term refers to the pathological state of excessive yin qi causing inhibition of physiological activities, excessive heat loss, and accumulation of pathogenic metabolites during disease development. While yin acts to cool, moisten, inhibit, and calm, pathogenic excess of yin featuring cold, inactivity, and dampness, with yang at a normal level, causes excess cold patterns. Clinically, it is manifested as cold body, cold limbs, lying curled up, pale and moist tongue, slow pulse, etc. Yin predominance giving rise to cold manifestations is mainly attributable to yin pathogenic factors such as cold-dampness, overconsumption of raw or cold foods, and cold retained in the middle energizer, rendering yang qi in the body unable to counter excessive yin. Thus yin qi becomes pathologically excessive.

【曾经译法】 an excess of *yin* brings about cold-syndrome; PREDOMINANT YIN PRODUCES COLD; Excess of *yin* may lead to cold; excess of yin leading to cold syndromes; Cold syndromes of excess type will occur in cases of excess of yin; Predominance of yin leads to cold syndrome; Exuberant yin brings about endogenous cold; Excessive Yin brings about Cold; excessive yin generating cold; hyper-yin generating cold

【现行译法】cold syndrome caused by an excess of yin; predominant yin leading to cold; predominance of yin leading to cold; abundance of yin producing cold manifestations; excessive yin giving rise to cold manifestations

【标准译法】Yin predominance causes cold.

【翻译说明】"阴胜则寒"中的"胜"表示偏胜，predominance 可表示在数量、局势上占优势或主导地位。"则"被译为 bring about, produce, lead to, occur, generate, cause 或 give rise to，都符合"则"表示"导致"的含义，其中 cause 和 give rise to 偏贬义，更符合原文语境；考虑到 cause 更简洁，所以选择 cause。

引例 Citations:

◎夫疟气者，并于阳则阳胜，并于阴则阴胜，阴胜则寒，阳胜则热。(《素问·疟论》)

（疟疾的邪气并入阳分，则使阳气胜；并入阴分，则使阴气胜。阴气偏盛就会产生寒象，阳气偏盛就会产生热象。）

When malarial qi merges into yang aspect, yang has predominance; when it merges into yin aspect, yin has predominance. Yin predominance causes cold manifestations, while yang predominance causes heat manifestations. (*Plain Conversation*)

◎或谓寒热者，阴阳争胜也，阳胜则热，阴胜则寒，此阴阳之争也。(《伤寒明理论》卷一)

（或者说感觉寒冷发热是因为阴阳争胜，阳气胜就发热，阴气胜就寒冷，这是阴阳相争的结果。）

In other words, chills and fever are the results of the struggle between yin and yang. Yin predominance causes cold manifestations, while yang predominance causes heat manifestations. (*Concise Exposition on Cold Damage*)

◎病有寒热者，由阴阳之有偏胜也。凡阳胜则热，以阴之衰也；阴胜则寒，以阳之衰也。（《景岳全书·杂证谟》）

> （疾病表现出恶寒发热的，是由于阴阳偏胜所致。凡是阳气偏盛就会产生热象，因为阴气的虚衰；阴气偏盛就会产生寒象，因为阳气的虚衰。）

Aversion to cold and fever are caused by the predominance of yin or yang. Yin predominance causes cold manifestations because of relative debilitation of yang; yang predominance causes heat manifestations because of relative debilitation of yin. (*Jingyue's Complete Works*) yángshèng zé rè

阳胜则热

Yang Predominance Causes Heat.

机体在疾病过程中，所出现的一种阳气病理性偏盛，功能亢奋，机体反应性增强，热量过剩的病理状态。阳气具有温煦、推动、兴奋等作用，阳气的病理性亢盛以热、动、燥为特点，形成阳盛而阴未虚的实热证，临床表现为壮热、烦渴、面红、目赤、尿黄、便干、苔黄、脉数等。导致阳胜则热的主要原因多是感受温热阳邪，或虽感受阴邪而从阳化热，也可由于情志内伤，五志过极而化火；或因气滞、血瘀、食积等郁而化热所致。

The term refers to the pathological state of excessive yang qi causing hyperactivity, increased body responsiveness, and excessive heat during disease development. While yang acts to warm, propel, and excite, its pathological excess, characterized by heat, hyperactivity, and dryness, with yin at a normal level, results in excess heat pattern. Clinically, it is manifested as high fever, vexation, thirst, redness of face and eyes, dark yellow urine, dry stool, yellowish tongue coating, rapid pulse, etc. Yang predominance giving rise to heat manifestations is mostly attributable to the attack by yang pathogenic factors such as warm-heat, the invasion by yin pathogenic factors which is transformed into heat, the damage from excessive emotions which turn into fire, and the heat resulting from depression due to qi stagnation, blood stasis, and food accumulation, etc.

【曾经译法】 An excess of *yang* brings about heat-syndrome; EXCESSIVE YANG PRODUCES HEAT; An excess of *yang* may bring about heat-syndrome; excess of yang leading to heat syndromes; Heat syndromes of excess type will occur in cases of excess of yang; Exuberance of yang leads to heat syndrome; Excess of Yang brings about Heat syndrome; excessive yang generating heat; hyper-yang generating heat

【现行译法】 heat syndrome due to an excess of yang; exuberance of yang generating heat; exuberant yang causing heat; heat syndrome brought about by extreme of yang; yang exuberance causing heat

【标准译法】 Yang predominance causes heat.

【翻译说明】 "阳胜则热"中的"胜"被译为 exuberance 和 excess 以及它们的形容词形式。此处与上一个词条保持一致，将"胜"译为 predominance。术语中的"则"表示因果关系。与其他类似词语相比，cause 偏向贬义语境，且最简练，因此选用。

引例 Citations:

◎病有寒热者，由阴阳之有偏胜也。凡阳胜则热，以阴之衰也；阴胜则寒，以阳之衰也。(《景岳全书·杂证谟》)

（疾病表现出恶寒发热的，是由于阴阳偏胜所致。凡是阳气偏盛就会产生热象，因为阴气的虚衰；阴气偏盛就会产生寒象，因为阳气的虚衰。）

Aversion to cold and fever are caused by the predominance of yin or yang. Yin predominance causes cold manifestations because of relative debilitation of yang; yang predominance causes heat manifestations because of relative debilitation of yin. (*Jingyue's Complete Works*)

◎阳胜则热，阴胜则寒，阴阳争则战。(《注解伤寒论》卷一)

（阳气偏盛就会产生热象，阴气偏盛就会产生寒象，阴阳相争就会战汗。）

Yin predominance causes cold manifestations, while yang predominance causes heat manifestations. The struggle between yin and yang leads to shivering and sweating at the same time. (*Annotated "Treatise on Cold Damage"*)

◎《经》曰阳胜则热，此为亢阳之火，证见烦渴燥结，小便赤涩，六脉洪数，治宜寒凉。（《医碥》卷一）

（《内经》说阳气偏盛就会产生热象，这是阳气亢盛之火，临床见心烦口渴，大便燥结，小便赤涩，六脉洪数，治疗宜用寒凉药物。）

According to *Yellow Emperor's Internal Canon of Medicine*, yang predominance may cause heat manifestations, which is the result of fire of excessive yang. Its clinical symptoms include vexation, thirst, dry stool, dark urine, difficult and painful urination, and surging rapid pulses on the six positions of the wrist. Herbal medicine cool or cold in property should be used for treatment. (*Stepping Stones for Medicine*) yīnsǔn jí yáng

阴损及阳

Yin Impairment Affects Yang.

由于阴精或阴气亏损，累及阳气生化不足，或阳气无所依附而耗散，从而在阴虚的基础上又出现了阳虚，进而形成了以阴虚为主的阴阳两虚的病理状态。例如肝阳上亢一证，其病机主要为肝肾阴虚，水不涵木，阴不制阳的阴虚阳亢，但病情发展，亦可进一步耗伤肝肾精血，影响肾阳化生，出现畏寒、肢冷、面色㿠白，脉沉细等肾阳虚衰的症状，转化为阴损及阳的阴阳两虚证。

The term refers to the pathological state characterized by primary yin deficiency and secondary yang deficiency. Deficiency or impairment of yin essence or yin qi affects the generation of yang qi, or leads to the consumption of yang qi as yin and yang are mutually dependent, resulting in yang deficiency in addition to yin deficiency. For example, the pattern of liver-yang hyperactivity is caused mainly by deficiency of both liver yin and kidney yin, which fails to control yang, or, in terms of the five elements, water fails to nourish wood. However, the disease may progress to impair blood and essence of the liver and the kidney, which would affect the generation and transformation of kidney yang and bring symptoms of kidney-yang deficiency such as aversion to cold, cold limbs, brightly pale complexion, and deep thready pulse. Thus, deficiency of both yin and yang occurs as a result of yin impairment affecting yang.

【曾经译法】 deficient *yin* affects *yang*; DEFICIENCY OF YIN AFFECTING YANG; *yang* involved by deficient *yin*; deficiency of yin affecting yang; impairment of yin affecting yang; Yin deficiency affects Yang; yin-consumption involving yang

【现行译法】 deficiency of yin affecting yang; impairment of yin involving yang; detriment of yin affecting yang; yin impairment involving yang; impairment of yin impeding generation of yang; impairment of

103

yin affecting yang; Detriment to yin affects yang; yin impairment affecting yang; syndrome/pattern of yin detriment affecting yang

【标准译法】Yin impairment affects yang.

【翻译说明】"损"不译为 deficiency，因为该词多用来翻译"虚"。相比 detriment，impairment 多指身心功能受损，更符合文意。术语中的"及"被译为 affect, involve 或 impede。其中，affect 表示"影响"，意思单一，偏贬义，符合原文意思；involve 意思较多，感情色彩偏中性；impede 表示"拖延、阻碍"，意思与原文不符。故"阴损及阳"译为 Yin impairment affects yang。

引例 Citations:

◎的是阴损及阳，而非六气客邪可通可泄，法当养胃之阴。(《临证指南医案》卷二)

（确实是阴气虚而损伤阳气，而不是六淫外感邪气，可以疏通、发泄，治法应当滋养胃阴。）

For cases caused by yin impairment affecting yang instead of six exogenous pathogenic factors, therapies of dredging and/or purgation could be used and stomach yin should be nourished. (*Case Records: A Guide to Clinical Practice*)

◎迩日形寒，不饥不欲食，缘阴损及阳。(《扫叶庄一瓢老人医案》卷一)

（近日形体寒冷，不饥不欲进食，是由于阴气虚而损伤阳气。）

The patient recently felt cold, and did not feel hungry with no desire to eat. This is a case of yin impairment affecting yang. (*Case Records of Elderly Yipiao in Saoye House*)

阳损及阴

Yang Impairment Affects Yin.

由于阳气虚损，无阳则阴无以生，从而在阳虚的基础上又导致了阴虚，形成以阳虚为主的阴阳两虚的病理状态。例如肾阳亏虚、水泛为肿一证，其病机主要为阳气不足，气化失司，水液代谢障碍，津液停聚而水湿内生，溢于肌肤。但其病变发展又可因阳气不足而导致阴气化生无源而亏虚，出现日益消瘦，甚则阳升风动而抽搐等肾阴亏虚之征象，转化为阳损及阴的阴阳两虚证。

The term refers to the pathological state characterized by primary yang deficiency and secondary yin deficiency. Deficiency or impairment of yang qi affects the generation of yin qi as yin and yang are mutually dependent, resulting in yin deficiency in addition to yang deficiency. For example, edema is caused mainly by deficiency of kidney yang. Deficient kidney yang fails to transform qi, which leads to disturbance of water metabolism and hence retention of body fluids in the skin. However, the disease may progress to deficiency of yin qi as deficient yang qi fails to generate sufficient yin qi and manifests symptoms of kidney-yin deficiency such as worsening emaciation and even convulsion as a result of stirring of wind due to ascending yang. Thus, deficiency of both yin and yang occurs as a result of yang impairment affecting yin.

【曾经译法】 Deficient *yang* affects *yin*; DEFICIENCY OF YANG AFFECTING YIN; *yin* involved by the deficient *yang*; weakness of yang affecting yin; impairment of yang affecting yin; Yang damages Yin; Deficiency of Yang affects Yin; yang-consumption involving yin

【现行译法】 deficiency of yang affecting yin; impairment of yang affecting yin; impairment of yang involving yin; yang impairment involving yin; impairment of yang impeding generation of yin; detriment to yang affects yin; yang impairment affecting yin; syndrome/pattern of yang detriment affecting yin

【标准译法】Yang impairment affects yin.

【翻译说明】"损"有 deficient, deficiency, weakness, impairment, damage, consumption 和 detriment 多种译法。其中，deficiency 指不足，多用于翻译"虚"；impairment 多指身体智力方面的障碍，也指功能损伤；weakness 可指系统、性格的缺陷；damage 强调造成物质方面的伤害；consumption 指能源、精力的损耗；detriment 指损害。"阳损及阴"中的"损"指阳气功能受损，impairment 比较合适。"及"的翻译有 affect, involve 和 impede 三种。其中，affect 表示"影响"，意思单一，偏贬义，比较符合原文意思；involve 意思较多，感情色彩偏中性；impede 表示"拖延、阻碍"，意思与原文不符。故"阳损及阴"译为 Yang impairment affects yin。

引例 Citations:

◎心衰乃阴损及阳，阳损及阴，阴阳并损，兼水饮痰浊为患。(《中国现代百名中医临床家丛书·石志超》)

Heart failure is caused by yin impairment affecting yang and yang impairment affecting yin, resulting in impairment of both yin and yang, accompanied with excessive retained morbid fluids and phlegm. (*100 Contemporary TCM Clinicians Series: Shi Zhichao*)

◎肾阳虚衰，阳损及阴，可导致阴阳两虚之证，甚至出现虚劳表现。(《中医病机辨证学》)

Kidney yang impairment affects yin and may lead to deficiency of both yin and yang, and even manifest as consumptive disease. (*Pattern Differentiation Based on Pathogenesis in Traditional Chinese Medicine*)

阳胜则阴病

Yang Predominance Causes Yin Disorder.

阳热偏胜导致各种伤津、伤阴的病理变化。阳盛之初，对阴气的损伤不明显，从而出现实热证。如果病情发展，阳热亢盛且明显耗伤机体阴气，疾病则从实热证转化为实热兼阴亏之象。若阳盛伤阴日久，阴气大伤，病可由实转虚而发展为虚热证。

The term refers to various pathological changes characterized by impairment of body fluids and yin due to predominance of yang heat. As yang becomes exuberant and its damage to yin is not yet obvious, excess heat pattern will occur. If the condition worsens, i.e., yang heat becomes increasingly excessive and causes obvious damage to yin in the body, the disease will progress from excess heat pattern to the pattern of excess heat accompanied with yin deficiency. In the long run, as yin might be damaged to a great extent, the disease may further develop from excess heat pattern into deficiency heat pattern.

【曾经译法】 an excess of *yang* leads to weakness of *yin*; EXCESS OF YANG CAUSING DISORDER OF YIN; An excess of *yang* leads to deficiency of *yin*; Predominance of Yang Consumes Yin; predominance of yang leading to disorder of yin; yang excess causing yin deficiency; hyper-yang causing hypo-yin

【现行译法】 disorder of yin caused by an excess of yang; exuberance of yang leading to disorder of yin; exuberant yang leading to disorder of yin; yang in excess making yin suffer; predominant yang making yin disorder; predominance of yang leading to disorder of yin

【标准译法】 Yang predominance causes yin disorder.

【翻译说明】 "阳胜则阴病"强调"阳胜"导致"阴病"。"阳胜"一般被译为 yang predominance。术语中的"则"表示因果关系，原因

"阳胜"在前时，翻译为 lead to, cause, consume 或 make，意思类似，但是 cause 最为简练，故选用。"病"译为 disorder，最贴近原文含义。

引例 Citations:

◎阴胜则阳病，阳胜则阴病。阳胜则热，阴胜则寒。（《素问·阴阳应象大论》）

（阴气偏盛，阳气就会受到损伤；阳气偏盛，阴气就会受到损伤。阳气偏盛就会产生热象，阴气偏盛就会产生寒象。）

Yin predominance causes yang disorder, giving rise to cold manifestations, while yang predominance causes yin disorder, giving rise to heat manifestations. (*Plain Conversation*)

◎阴盛则阳亏，阳盛则阴亏，所谓阳胜则阴病，阴胜则阳病。（《活人事证方后集》卷十五）

（阴气偏盛就会使阳气亏虚，阳气偏盛就会使阴气亏虚，所谓阳气偏盛，阴气就会受到损伤；阴气偏盛，阳气就会受到损伤。）

Yin predominance leads to yang deficiency, and yang predominance leads to yin deficiency. In other words, yin predominance causes yang disorder and yang predominance causes yin disorder. (*Formulas for Pattern Treatment to Safeguard Life*) yīnshèng zé yángbìng

阴胜则阳病

Yin Predominance Causes Yang Disorder.

阴寒偏胜导致阳气衰微的病理变化。阴寒内盛，日久则必损伤阳气，故常伴有机体生理功能减退，阳热不足的阳虚征象，出现实寒兼阳虚之象。若阴盛伤阳日久，阳气损伤严重，病可由实转虚而发展为虚寒证。

The term refers to the pathological change of yang-qi decline caused by predominance of yin cold. Excessive yin cold in the body will impair yang qi in the long run, causing yang deficiency characterized by a decrease in physiological functions of the body and insufficiency of yang heat. Thus, symptoms of both excess cold and yang deficiency manifest themselves. If yin predominance has damaged yang for a long time, yang qi will be seriously impaired, and the disease may progress from an excess pattern to a deficiency cold pattern.

【曾经译法】 An excess of *yin* leads to weakness of *yang*; EXCESS OF YIN CAUSING DISORDER OF YANG; An excess of *yin* leads to deficiency of *yang*; Predominance of Yin Consumes Yang; Predominant yin leads to disorder of yang; Excess of Yin leads to disorder of Yang; yin excess causing yang deficiency; hyper-yin causing hypo-yang

【现行译法】 disorder of yang due to an excess of yin; predominant yin leading to yang disease; yin in excess making yang suffer; excessive yin making yang suffer; predominant yin making yang disorder; predominance of yin leading to disorder of yang

【标准译法】 Yin predominance causes yang disorder.

【翻译说明】 "阴胜则阳病"强调"阴胜"导致"阳病"。"阴胜"一般被译为 yin predominance。术语中的"则"表示因果关系，原因"阴胜"在前时，翻译为 lead to, cause 和 make，意思类似，但是 cause 偏向贬义语境，故选用。"病"译为 disorder 最贴近原文含义。

引例 Citations:

◎阳不足则阴乘之，其变为寒。故阴胜则阳病，阴胜为寒也。（《景岳全书·传忠录》）

（阳气不足就会使阴气相对偏盛，病变呈现寒象。因此阴气偏盛就会使阳气亏虚，阴气偏盛就会产生寒象。）

Deficiency of yang qi will make yin relatively excessive, and cold signs and symptoms may occur. Therefore, yin predominance causes yang disorder and cold manifestations occur. (*Jingyue's Complete Works*)

◎阴病则血留之而阴胜，阴胜则阳病矣。（《医经原旨》卷五）

（阴分有病就会使血液留滞而导致阴偏盛，阴气偏盛，阳气就会受到损伤。）

Pathological changes of yin will lead to blood stasis, which causes predominance of yin. Yin predominance may cause yang disorder. (*Original Decrees of Medicine*)

阴盛格阳

Exuberant Yin Repels Yang.

阴盛格阳又称格阳，系指阴寒偏盛至极，壅闭于内，逼迫阳气浮越于外的一种病理状态。阴寒内盛是疾病的本质，由于排斥阳气于外，可在原有面色苍白、四肢逆冷、精神萎靡、脉微欲绝等阴气偏盛于内表现的基础上，又出现面红、烦热、口渴、脉大无根等假热之象，故称其为真寒假热证。另外，临床上还有一种称为"戴阳"的病变，是指下元真阳极度虚弱，阳不制阴，偏盛之阴盘踞于内，逼迫衰极之阳浮越于上，阴阳不相维系的一种下真寒、上假热的病变，亦属于阴盛格阳。

The term, also known as repelling yang, refers to the pathological state in which extremely exuberant yin cold is congested inside the body, forcing yang qi to flow to the body surface. Excessive internal yin cold is the fundamental cause of the disease. However, as yang qi is repelled by yin cold and driven to the body surface, pseudo-heat symptoms may appear such as red face, vexing heat, thirst, and apparently surging pulse without root in addition to the original symptoms of excessive yin in the interior such as pale complexion, reversal cold of the limbs, listlessness, and feeble pulse. Thus, it is described as the pattern of true cold with pseudo-heat. Clinically, a disease known as "floating yang" is also a manifestation of exuberant yin repelling yang. It is characterized by lower cold in nature and upper heat in disguise as a result of the failure of yin and yang to maintain each other when true yang (kidney qi) is extremely weak and fails to restrict yin and yin becomes excessive in the body and drives the feeble yang to the upper part of the body.

【曾经译法】 *Yang* is kept externally by the excessive *yin* inside the body; EXCESSIVE YIN HINDERS YANG; excessive *yin* repelling yang; exuberant yin repelling yang; Excessive Yin keeps Yang externally; excessive yin rejecting yang

【现行译法】yang kept externally by yin excess in the interior; predominant yin rejecting yang; exuberant yin repelling yang; excessive yin repelling yang; pseudo-heat manifestations in the exterior due to extreme cold in the interior; syndrome/pattern of exuberant yin with repelled yang

【标准译法】Exuberant yin repels yang.

【翻译说明】"盛" 被译为 excessive, excess, exuberant, predominant 和 extreme。其中, exuberant（abounding, 大量存在, 有许多）较为常用, 世界中医药学会联合会标准等也采用这一译法。动词 "格" 表示格拒, 译为 repel 意思较准确, 具有动态, 并且简洁。

引例 Citations:

◎伤寒阴盛格阳者, 病人身冷, 脉细沉疾, 烦躁而不饮者是也。(《阴证略例》)

（伤寒病阴盛格阳, 临床表现为病人感觉身冷, 脉象细沉数疾, 烦躁而不欲饮水。）

Patients who suffer from cold damage with exuberant yin repelling yang are found to have cold sensation, thready deep rapid or racing pulse, vexation, and no desire to drink water. (*Brief Cases of Yin Pattern*)

◎假热者, 水极似火, 阴证似阳也……亦曰阴盛格阳也。(《叶选医衡》)

（假热证, 水盛极而好像火, 阴证好像阳证……也称之为阴盛格阳。）

In the cases of pseudo-heat pattern, water becomes extremely excessive, like fire, making yin pattern appear like yang pattern... It is also described as exuberant yin repelling yang. (*Ye's Medical Measures*)

◎伤寒未三日，身冷，额上汗出，面赤心烦者，非阴毒证，谓之阴盛格阳。（《脉因证治》卷一）

> （患伤寒病没有三天，身体冷，额头出汗，面赤，心烦，这不是阴毒证，而是阴盛格阳。）

If a patient has had cold damage for less than three days and feels cold with sweat on the forehead, redness of face, and vexation, it is not a case of yin-toxin pattern, but exuberant yin repelling yang. (*Symptoms, Causes, Pulses, and Treatments*) yángshèng géyīn

阳盛格阴

Exuberant Yang Repels Yin.

阳盛格阴又称格阴，系指阳热偏盛至极，深伏于里，阳气被遏，郁闭于内，不能外达而将阴气排斥于外的一种病理状态。阳盛于内是疾病的本质，但由于格阴于外，可在原有壮热、面红、气粗、烦躁、舌红、脉数大有力等邪热内盛表现的基础上，又出现四肢厥冷、脉象沉伏等假寒之象，故称为真热假寒证。

The term, also known as repelling yin, refers to the pathological state in which extremely exuberant yang heat is hidden deeply inside the body, or in other words, yang qi is obstructed inside the body and fails to flow to the body surface while yin qi is driven out. Exuberant yang in the interior is the fundamental cause of the disease. However, as yin qi is repelled by yang heat and driven to the body surface, symptoms of pseudo-cold such as reversal cold of the limbs as well as deep hidden pulse may appear in addition to the original symptoms of excessive heat pathogen in the interior such as high fever, redness of face, heavy breathing, vexation, red tongue, and forceful rapid surging pulse. Thus, it is called the pattern of true heat with pseudo-cold.

【曾经译法】 *Yin* is kept externally by the excessive *yang* inside the body; EXCESSIVE YANG HINDERS YIN; *Yin* is kept superficially by excessive *yang* inside body; Exuberant yang repels yin; Excessive Yang keeps Yin externally; excessive yang rejecting yin

【现行译法】 yin kept externally by yang excess in the interior; exuberant yang repelling yin; superabundant yang rejecting yin; pseudo-cold manifestations in the exterior due to extreme heat in the interior

【标准译法】 Exuberant yang repels yin.

【翻译说明】 " 盛 " 被 译 为 excessive, excess, exuberant, superabundant 或

extreme，与上一词条保持一致，采用 exuberant。动词"格"表示格拒，译为 repel 意思准确，具有动态，并且简洁。

引例 Citations:

◎至若假寒者，火极似水，阳证似阴也……亦日阳盛格阴也。(《叶选医衡》)

（至于假寒证，火盛极好像水，阳证好像阴证……也称之为阳盛格阴。）

In the cases of pseudo-cold pattern, fire becomes extremely excessive, like water, making yang pattern appear like yin pattern... It is also described as exuberant yang repelling yin. (*Ye's Medical Measures*)

◎阳盛拒阴，身表凉痛，四脚冷，诸阴证，脉沉数而有力，承气主之。(《脉因证治》卷一)

（阳盛拒阴，体表寒凉疼痛，四肢冷，表现类似阴证，但脉沉数有力，用承气汤类主治。）

Exuberant yang repelling yin causes a pattern like that of yin, manifested as cold pain in the body surface, cold limbs, but forceful deep rapid pulse. It is an indication for *Chengqi* Decoction (Decoction for Purging Digestive Qi). (*Symptoms, Causes, Pulses, and Treatments*)

◎若温病恶寒，口燥咽干，舌黄唇焦，乃阳盛格阴，内热则外寒，非恶寒也。(《伤寒瘟疫条辨》卷二)

（若温病出现恶寒，但口燥咽干，舌黄唇焦，这是阳盛格阴，内有实热而外有寒象，并不是恶寒。）

In the cases of febrile diseases, if aversion to cold occurs but with dry mouth and throat, yellowish tongue, and chapped lips, it is the manifestation of exuberant yang repelling yin, i.e., there is excess heat in the interior with cold signs and symptoms in the exterior. It is not truly aversion to cold. (*Systematic Differentiation of Cold Damage and Warm Epidemics*)

阳微阴弦

Faint Pulse at Yang and Wiry Pulse at Yin

脉象寸部脉微而尺部脉弦，是从脉象上说明胸痹与心痛的病机。寸脉为阳，尺脉为阴。寸部脉见微弱之象，说明上焦阳气不足，胸阳不振。尺部脉见弦象，说明阴寒邪盛，水饮内停。"阳微"与"阴弦"并见，说明胸痹、心痛的病机是上焦阳虚，阴邪上乘，邪正相搏而成。《金匮要略·胸痹心痛短气病脉证治》说："今阳虚知在上焦，所以胸痹、心痛者，以其阴弦故也。"进一步指出"阳微"与"阴弦"是胸痹、心痛病因病机不可缺少的两个方面。

The term refers to faint pulse at the *cun* (寸) section and wiry pulse at the *chi* (尺) section, the pulse manifestations of chest impediment and heart pain from the perspective of pathogenesis. Pulse at the *cun* section is yang, while pulse at the *chi* section is yin. The faint pulse at the *cun* section indicates insufficiency of yang qi in the upper energizer and hypofunction of yang qi in the chest. The wiry pulse at the *chi* section shows yin-cold excess and water retention. The concurrence of the two pulse manifestations indicates that chest impediment and heart pain are caused by yang deficiency in the upper energizer leading to the attack of the upper energizer by yin pathogens and fight between pathogenic qi and healthy qi. According to the section "Pulses, Patterns, and Treatments of Diseases of Chest Impediment, Heart Pain, and Shortness of Breath" in *Essential Prescriptions of the Golden Cabinet,* "Now through examination, it is known that yang deficiency exists in the upper energizer. The chest impediment and heart pain are attributable to the fight between yin and yang as is indicated by wiry pulse at yin (the *chi* section)." This further illustrates that the manifestations of faint pulse at yang and wiry pulse at yin are indispensable aspects of the etiology and pathogenesis of chest impediment and heart pain.

【曾经译法】 /

【现行译法】 weak pulse at yang and wiry pulse at yin

【标准译法】 faint pulse at yang and wiry pulse at yin

【翻译说明】 "阳微阴弦"的"阳"指的是寸口处的脉，译为 pulse at yang
意思准确、简练。与 weak 相比，faint 指影像、气味或者声
音等几乎觉察不到，符合语境。译词 wiry 指头发等的外形或
触感像铁丝一样细而硬，意思更贴近原文。

引例 Citations:

◎夫脉当取太过不及，阳微阴弦，即胸痹而痛，所以然者，责其极虚也。
(《金匮要略·胸痹心痛短气病脉证治》)

（诊脉首先应当注意太过与不及，寸部脉微而尺部脉弦，主胸痹、
心痛。所以如此，关键在于阳气极虚。）

Pay attention to excess and insufficiency when taking pulse. Faint pulse at
yang (the *cun* section) and wiry pulse at yin (the *chi* section) indicates chest
impediment and heart pain. The underlying cause is that yang qi is extremely
weak. (*Essential Prescriptions of the Golden Cabinet*)

◎胸痹之脉，阳微阴弦，阳微知在上焦，阴弦则为心痛，此《金匮》《千
金》均以通阳主治也。(《类证治裁》)

（胸痹的脉象，寸部脉微而尺部脉弦，由寸部脉微知其病在上焦，
尺部脉弦就会出现心痛。这就是《金匮要略》《千金要方》都采
用通阳法治疗的原因。）

The pulse manifestation of chest impediment is faint pulse at yang and wiry
pulse at yin. Faint pulse at yang means the disease is in the upper energizer,
and wiry pulse at yin means heart pain may appear. Hence, the therapy of
unblocking yang should be adopted according to *Essential Prescriptions of
the Golden Cabinet* and *Important Formulas Worth a Thousand Gold Pieces*.
(*Categorized Patterns with Clear-cut Treatments*)

◎所云寸口脉沉而迟，阳微阴弦，是知但有寒症而无热症矣。（《临证指南医案》卷四）

（所言寸口脉沉而迟，寸部脉微而尺部脉弦，由此可知只有寒证而没有热证。）

Deep slow radial pulse as well as faint pulse at yang and wiry pulse at yin indicates a case of cold pattern, not heat pattern. (*Case Records: A Guide to Clinical Practice*) qìjī shītiáo

气机失调

Qi Movement Disorder

气的运行不畅或升降出入运动失去平衡协调的病理变化。中医学认为气的运动正常表现在两方面，一是气的运动必须通畅无阻，二是气的升降出入运动之间必须协调平衡。这种状态称为气机调畅，反之则为气机失调。由于气的运动形式的多样性，所以气机失调也有多种表现：气滞是指气的运行不畅，郁阻停滞，以胀闷、疼痛为特征；气逆指气的升发太过或下降不及，以肺、胃、肝等脏腑病变最为多见；气陷指气的上升不足或下降太过，主要以气虚升举无力而下陷为特征；气闭指气机郁闭，外出受阻，导致清窍闭塞，以突然昏厥、不省人事为特点；气脱指气不内守，大量外逸，以致全身功能突然衰竭的病理变化。

The term refers to the pathological changes of inhibited qi flow or uncoordinated and imbalanced ascending, descending, exiting, and entering of qi. According to traditional Chinese medicine, normal movement of qi should be smooth, unimpeded, coordinated, and balanced; otherwise, it is known as qi movement disorder. Due to the diversity of qi movement, there are various manifestations of qi movement disorder. For example, qi stagnation means the movement of qi is obstructed, constrained, inhibited, and stagnated, resulting in distention, oppression, and pain. Qi counterflow refers to excessive ascending or insufficient descending of qi, mostly causing pathological changes of the lung, the stomach, the liver and other zang-fu organs. Qi sinking refers to inadequate ascending or excessive descending of qi, marked by sinking of qi as qi is deficient and unable to lift. Qi block means that qi movement is constrained and blocked, and qi fails to exit, leading to the obstruction of clear orifices, featured by fainting and unconsciousness. Qi collapse means that qi fails to stay inside the body and flows outside in large amounts, resulting in a sudden complete failure of body functions.

【曾经译法】 /

【现行译法】 disorder of qi movement; qi movement disorder

【标准译法】 qi movement disorder

【翻译说明】分析"气机失调"的现行译法,"气机"一词均译为 qi movement,而"失调"均译为 disorder,较为准确。出于简洁性和回译性考虑,选用 qi movement disorder。

引例 Citations:

◎人参散,治五噎,胃脘气滞,心胸满闷,咽喉中噎塞,气机不运,不能下食。(《普济方》卷二百五)

（人参散,治疗五种噎证,胃脘气滞,心胸满闷,咽喉中堵塞,气机不能运行,不能进食。）

Renshen Powder (Ginseng Powder) is used to treat five kinds of dysphagia, namely, qi stagnation in gastric cavity, fullness and oppression in the heart and chest, obstruction in the throat, disorder of qi movement, and inability to eat. (*Formulas for Universal Relief*)

◎秽湿着里,舌黄脘闷,气机不宣,久则酿热,三加减正气散主之。(《温病条辨》卷二)

（秽湿之邪留着于内,舌苔黄,胃脘胀闷,气机不畅,日久就生热,用三加减正气散主治。）

As filth and dampness remain inside the body, yellowish tongue coating, gastric distension and fullness, as well as qi movement disorder occur. Over time, heat is generated. The Third Variant *Zheng Qi* Powder (Qi-correcting Powder) should be used. (*Systematic Differentiation of Warm Diseases*) yíngwèi bùhé

营卫不和

Nutrient-defense Disharmony

营气与卫气不能协调的病理现象。营，即营气，主内守而属阴；卫，即卫气，主卫外而属阳。在生理状态下，卫行脉外，具有护卫肌表，温养肌肉、皮毛，以及调节控制腠理的开合、汗液的排泄等功能；营行脉中，能够营养濡润脏腑及四肢百骸。营卫相互协调，是维护人体正常功能，不受外邪侵袭致病的重要前提。若形体虚弱，或外感风邪，营卫之气失于和调，则阳气卫外不固，阴液易于外泄，可出现时时发热、自汗、怕冷或畏风等症状。在外感风邪或内伤杂病中均可见到。

The term refers to the disharmony between nutrient qi and defense qi. Nutrient qi or nutrient corresponds to yin and stays in the interior, and defense qi or defense corresponds to yang and defends in the exterior. In physiological state, defense qi, which flows outside the vessels, protects fleshy exterior and warms as well as nourishes muscles, skin, and body hair. It also regulates and controls the opening and closing of striae and interstices as well as the excretion of sweat, etc. Nutrient qi, which flows inside the vessels, nourishes and moistens the zang-fu organs, limbs, and skeleton. Harmony and coordination between nutrient qi and defense qi is an important prerequisite for normal function of human body and defense against external pathogens. If the body is weak, or externally contracts wind pathogen, disharmony between nutrient qi and defense qi will occur. As a result, yang qi fails to secure the exterior and yin fluids tend to be excreted easily, resulting in symptoms such as fever, spontaneous sweating, and fear of cold or wind. Nutrient-defense disharmony can be found in cases of external contraction of wind pathogen or miscellaneous internal diseases.

【曾经译法】imbalance between *ying*-energy and *wei*-energy; DISHARMONY BETWEEN YING (NUTRIENTS) AND WEI (DEFENSE MECHANISM); derangement between nutrient and defensive qi; disharmony between nutrient qi and defensive qi; disharmony between nutrient Qi and defensive Qi

【现行译法】disharmony between nutritive-qi and defensive-qi; disharmony between ying qi and wei qi; disharmony between nutrient qi and defensive qi; disharmony between nutrient and defense; disharmony between ying and wei systems; disharmony between nutrient and defense (systems); nutrient-defense disharmony; disharmony between nutrient and defensive qi; syndrome/pattern of nutrient qi and defense qi disharmony

【标准译法】nutrient-defense disharmony

【翻译说明】从意思上看，nutrient（具有营养作用的物质）和 defense（具有保卫作用的事物）较为准确、简练，能与中文术语中的"营""卫"字面和意思基本对应。"不和"被译为 imbalance，disharmony 和 derangement。译词 disharmony 指若干元素发生冲突，无法形成具有一致性的整体；imbalance 指对应事物之间比例失调或缺少关联；derangement 指功能失常紊乱。从意思上看，disharmony 最为适合。从术语结构角度分析，加上连字符的 nutrient-defense disharmony 最为精炼。

引例 Citations:

◎设见脉浮，自汗，营卫不和，纵非外感，仍属桂枝汤证矣。（《伤寒缵论》卷下）

（假若出现脉浮，自汗，营卫之气不相协调，即使不是外感疾病，仍然属于桂枝汤证。）

Even if such symptoms of nutrient-defense disharmony as floating pulse and spontaneous sweating do not fall into the cases of externally contracted disease, they are still indications for *Guizhi* Decoction (Cinnamon Twig Decoction). (*Continued Treatise on Cold Damage*)

◎未有营卫不和而脉能通者，故以芍药、甘草、大枣调和营卫。（《成方切用》卷六）

    （没有营卫之气不相协调而脉道能够通畅的，所以用芍药、甘草、大枣以调和营卫。）

In cases of nutrient-defense disharmony, vessels must have been obstructed, so *shaoyao* (*Radix Paeoniae Alba seu Rubra*, white or red peony root), *gancao* (*Radix et Rhizoma Glycyrrhizae*, licorice root), and *dazao* (*Fructus Jujubae*, Chinese date) should be used to harmonize nutrient and defense aspects. (*Effective Use of Established Formulas*)

◎气凝血滞，而营卫不和，经水先后多寡不一也。（《医旨绪余》卷下）

    （气血凝滞不畅，而营卫之气不相协调，月经来潮先后、多少不一致。）

The stagnation of qi and blood, together with nutrient-defense disharmony, leads to irregular periods in timing and/or quantity. (*Remnants of Medical Decree*)

营弱卫强

Weak Nutrient and Strong Defense

太阳中风证卫阳浮越外泄，营阴不能内守的病机。风为阳邪，伤于卫表。风邪外袭时，人体卫阳的升散性、动性占优势，阳气外浮与邪相争则发热；风为阳邪，其性开泄，以致卫不外固，营不内守则自汗出；汗出而肌腠疏松，不胜风邪，故恶风；营阴不足，加之风性散漫，故脉来浮缓。故太阳中风证以发热恶风、自汗出、脉浮缓为主症。

The term refers to the pathogenesis of *taiyang* (greater yang) wind-invasion pattern, i.e., defense yang floats outside and nutrient yin fails to stay inside the body. Wind is a yang pathogen and attacks the defense exterior. When pathogenic wind invades, defense qi, which ascends, dissipates, and moves, floats out to body surface to fight against the wind pathogen, resulting in fever. Being opening and dispersing, the pathogenic wind makes the defense exterior become insecure and fail to keep nutrient qi in the interior, resulting in spontaneous sweating. As interstitial space enlarges and muscles relax with perspiration, human body cannot defend against the wind pathogen, and aversion to wind may occur. Due to the weakness of nutrient qi and the dispersing nature of wind, the pulse of the patient is floating and moderate. In sum, the main symptoms of *taiyang* wind-invasion pattern include fever, aversion to wind, spontaneous sweating, and floating moderate pulse.

【曾经译法】 /

【现行译法】 weakness of nutritive-qi and hyper-activities of the defensive qi; strong defense with weak nutrient (卫强营弱); excess of defense qi and deficiency of nutrient qi (卫强营弱)

【标准译法】 weak nutrient and strong defense

【翻译说明】 此处"营弱"指的是营气由于风邪性开泄而不内守，表现相对虚弱，而"卫强"指的是卫气为抵御风邪而活跃于肌表，表现相对强盛，所以二者关系为并列关系，应该使用连词 and。"营弱卫强"指的是营阴较弱，卫气占优势，而不是营气不足，卫气过多，因此不用 deficiency（缺少）和 excess（超过），而选用 weak 和 strong。

引例 Citations:

◎太阳病，发热汗出者，此为营弱卫强，故使汗出，欲救邪风者，宜桂枝汤。（《伤寒论》）

（太阳病表现为发热汗出的，这是卫阳浮越外泄，营阴不能内守，所以使人体汗出。欲救治风邪所伤的病证，宜用桂枝汤。）

Taiyang disease characterized by fever and perspiration indicates weak nutrient and strong defense. That is why there is perspiration. The appropriate formula for treating diseases caused by wind pathogen is *Guizhi* Decoction (Cinnamon Twig Decoction). (*Treatise on Cold Damage*)

◎此即申明上条"阳浮者热自发，阴弱者汗自出"，由营弱卫强故也。弱者因津液走泄而弱，强者因风邪鼓动而强。（《医门棒喝》卷二）

（这是申明上一条"阳浮者热自发，阴弱者汗自出"，是因为卫阳浮越外泄，营阴不能内守所致。弱者是因为津液外泄而营弱，强者是因为风邪鼓动而卫强。）

This is to explain the quotation of "floating defense yang resulting in fever and weak nutrient yin resulting in perspiration" in the previous article. It means such symptoms are caused by weak nutrient and strong defense. Nutrient qi becomes weaker due to the loss of body fluids, while defense qi becomes stronger due to the invasion of pathogenic wind. (*Medical Warnings*) yíngqiáng wèiruò

营强卫弱

Strong Nutrient and Weak Defense

太阳伤寒证指营阴郁滞，卫阳被遏的病机。寒为阴邪，易伤营阴。感受寒邪时，人体营阴的沉降性、静性增强而跃居优势，卫阳被郁于肤表之内，不得发散于外以温煦肤表，故恶寒；阳气郁遏于内不得宣散则发热；寒邪外束，毛窍闭塞，则无汗、脉浮紧；营卫不和，经络不畅，则头项强痛，骨节疼痛。故太阳表实证以发热恶寒、无汗、头项强痛、骨节疼痛、脉浮紧为主症。

The term refers to the pathogenesis of *taiyang* cold-damage pattern, i.e., nutrient yin is constrained and defense yang obstructed. Cold is a yin pathogen and is prone to attack nutrient yin. When pathogenic cold invades, nutrient qi, due to its increase in descent and inactivity, obstructs the defense qi in the interior, making defense qi unable to disperse on body surface to warm the skin, and thus aversion to cold occurs. When yang qi is obstructed inside and unable to disperse, fever also occurs. Moreover, when pathogenic cold fetters the exterior and blocks the pores, absence of sweating and floating tight pulse could be found. Finally, defense-nutrient disharmony and obstructed meridians and collaterals could result in headache, painful stiff nape, and painful joints. In sum, the main symptoms of *taiyang* exterior excess pattern include fever, aversion to cold, absence of sweating, headache, painful stiff nape, painful joints, and floating tight pulse.

【曾经译法】/

【现行译法】weak defense with strong nutrient (卫弱营强); weak defense qi and strong nutrient (卫弱营强); deficiency of defense qi and excess of nutrient qi (卫弱营强)

【标准译法】strong nutrient and weak defense

【翻译说明】"营阴"因郁滞，表现相对强盛，而"卫阳"因被遏，表现相对虚弱，二者关系为并列关系，应该使用连词 and。"营强卫弱"指的是营气占优势，卫阳被遏，而不是营气过多，卫气缺少，因此不用 excess（超过）和 deficiency（缺少），而用 strong 和 weak 表示程度。

引例 Citations:

◎寒并于营，营实而卫虚者，无汗而恶风也，以营强卫弱。(《伤寒纪玄妙用集》卷二)

（寒邪侵入营分，营分实而卫分虚的，表现为无汗而怕风，这是因为营阴郁滞，卫阳被遏。）

As pathogenic cold invades nutrient aspect, excess pattern of nutrient aspect and deficiency pattern of defense aspect would be found. The symptoms include absence of sweating and aversion to wind as a result of strong nutrient (due to stagnation) and weak defense (due to being constrained). (*Profound Significance and Ingenious Uses of the "Treatise on Cold Damage"*)

◎以营强卫弱，故气逆而喘，与麻黄汤，以发其汗。(《伤寒直指》)

（由于营阴郁滞，卫阳被遏，所以气上逆而喘息，用麻黄汤发汗治疗。）

Mahuang Decoction (Ephedra Decoction) which induces sweating should be used to relieve panting caused by ascending counterflow of qi due to strong nutrient and weak defense. (*Direct Guidance on Cold Damage*) wǔzhì huà huǒ

五志化火

Five Emotions Transform into Fire.

怒、喜、思、悲、恐五种情志太过，郁久生热化火的病理变化。五志化火，又称"五志过极化火"，是由于精神情志刺激，影响脏腑精气阴阳的协调平衡，导致脏腑阳盛亢逆，或气机郁结，气郁日久而从阳化火所形成的病理改变。如情志内伤，抑郁不畅，则常能导致肝郁气滞，气郁化火，或大怒伤肝，肝气亢逆化火，均可发为肝火。

The term refers to the pathological change caused by excess of five emotions and mental activities, namely, anger, joy, overthinking, sorrow, and fear. In the long run, they generate heat and transform into fire. "Five emotions transforming into fire" or "the excess of five emotions transforming into fire" refers to the pathological changes caused by mental and emotional overstimulation, which affects coordination and balance of the zang-fu organs, essential qi, and yin and yang, leading to yang excess, hyperactivity, and counterflow in zang-fu organs, or causes constraint and stagnation of qi, transforming into yang and fire if such qi constraint and stagnation lasts for a long time. For instance, internal damage caused by uncontrolled emotions and depression often lead to liver qi constraint and stagnation, which then transforms into liver fire. Another example is that anger damages the liver, leading to hyperactivity and counterflow of liver qi, which may transform into liver fire.

【曾经译法】 fire-syndrome caused by the disorders of the five emotions; FIVE EMOTIONS PRODUCING FIRE; fire-syndrome caused by the disorders of five emotions; five emotions transforming into fire; Five excessive emotions convert into internal Fire

【现行译法】 heat syndromes caused by the disorders of five emotions; five emotions transforming into fire; fire syndrome triggered by emotional stress; transformation of five emotions into fire;

transformation of the five minds into fire; five minds transforming into fire

【标准译法】Five emotions transform into fire.

【翻译说明】"五志"指的是怒、喜、思、悲、恐五种情志，多译为 five emotions，较为准确简练。"化"多译为 transform into 的动词或者名词形式，或译为 cause, produce, trigger, convert into，其中 transform into 意思最为准确，强调转化。故"五志化火"译为 Five emotions transform into fire。

引例 Citations:

◎河间有曰：五志过极皆为火也。(《丹溪心法》卷十四)

（刘河间曾说：五志过极皆可化为火。）

Liu Hejian once said that excessive five emotions can transform into fire. (*Danxi's Mastery of Medicine*)

◎因烦劳则五志过极，动火而卒中，皆因热甚生火。(《临证指南医案》卷一)

（因为烦劳导致五种情志太过，化火而发生中风，都是因为热极而产生火。）

Vexation and overstrain may lead to excessive five emotions, which may transform into fire and result in stroke. The pathogenesis is that extreme heat produces fire. (*Case Records: A Guide to Clinical Practice*)

◎亦有因五志有所过极而卒中者，夫五志过极皆为热甚，俗云风者，言末而忘其本也。(《张氏医通》卷一)

（也有因为五种情志太过而患中风的，五种情志太过都导致内热严重，一般认为是风的，是看到表象而忘记其根本了。）

In addition, some patients suffer from stroke because of excessive five emotions which can transform into intense internal heat. Those who believe that such stroke is caused by wind only see the branch and forget the root. (*Comprehensive Medicine by Doctor Zhang Lu*)

肝阳化风

Liver Yang Transforms into Wind.

肝肾阴亏，水不涵木，肝阳亢逆无制而动风的病理变化。肝阳化风多由于情志所伤，郁而化火，郁火伤阴，或操劳过度，耗伤肝肾之阴，以致阴虚阳亢，肝阳浮动不潜，亢逆化风，形成风动之势。临床可见眩晕欲仆，筋惕肉𥆧，肢麻震颤，口眼㖞斜，或半身不遂，甚则血随气逆而猝然仆倒，或为闭厥，或为脱厥。肝阳化风以中风病为多见。

The term refers to the pathological change due to depletion of liver yin and kidney yin, in which the kidney (water) fails to nourish the liver (wood), and thus, hyperactivity and counterflow of liver yang without restriction stir wind. In most cases, liver yang transforming into wind is due to the constraint of emotions which causes internal damage and transforms into fire, and hence damages yin. Another possibility is that overstrain consumes and damages liver yin and kidney yin, causing yin deficiency and yang hyperactivity. Thus, liver yang floats and cannot be subdued, whose hyperactivity and counterflow transform into stirring wind. Clinically, it is manifested as dizziness, proneness to forward fall, muscle twitching, limb numbness and tremor, facial palsy, or hemiplegia. In severe cases, sudden forward fall may occur due to the counterflow of qi and blood such as wind-stroke block and wind-stroke collapse. Liver yang transforming into wind is often seen in the cases of wind-stroke.

【曾经译法】 Liver-Yang changes into Liver-Wind.

【现行译法】 interior wind caused by excessive liver-yang; liver-yang transforming into wind; transformation of liver yang into wind; syndrome/pattern of liver yang transforming into wind

【标准译法】 Liver yang transforms into wind.

【翻译说明】"肝阳"多译为 liver yang，准确简练，与原文对应。"化"多译为 transform into 及其名词形式，在意思和语法上都比较准确。故"肝阳化风"译为 Liver yang transforms into wind。

引例 Citations:

◎上升之气自肝而出，中挟相火，故气病多属肝逆犯胃，肝阳化风。（《类证治裁》卷三）

（上逆的气从肝发出，其中夹有相火，所以气病大多属于肝气逆而犯胃，肝阳亢盛化风。）

Ascending counterflow of qi from the liver carries ministerial fire with it, so most qi-related diseases manifest the pathogenesis of counterflow of liver qi invading the stomach or hyperactive liver yang transforming into wind. (*Categorized Patterns with Clear-cut Treatments*)

◎诊脉左劲右濡，据症是水弱木失滋涵，肝阳化风。（《临证指南医案》卷三）

（诊脉左手劲急，右手浮而细软，据此判断是肾阴不足，肝木失于滋养，肝阳亢盛化风。）

Racing pulse at the left hand of the patient and soggy pulse at the right hand indicates kidney-yin deficiency, which fails to nourish and moisten the liver, and thus, liver yang becomes hyperactive and transforms into wind. (*Case Records: A Guide to Clinical Practice*)

◎肝阳化风，逆行脾胃之分，液聚成痰，流走肝胆之络。（《静香楼医案》）

（肝阳亢盛化风，横逆影响脾胃，脾胃运化失常，水湿不运聚集成痰，流走于肝胆络脉。）

Hyperactive liver yang transforms into wind, its transverse invasion affecting the spleen and the stomach, leading to transportation and transformation disorder. As a result, water-dampness that has not been transported away accumulates to form phlegm, which flows in the collaterals of the liver and the gallbladder. (*Case Records of Jingxiang Mansion*)

阴虚生风

Yin Deficiency Generates Wind.

肝肾阴液枯竭，筋脉失养而风气内动的病理变化。阴虚生风多因热病后期，阴液不足，或久病耗阴，或因年迈肝肾之阴自然亏耗，阴液不足，不能滋养濡润筋脉而变生内风。临床可见手足蠕动、筋惕肉瞤等，并伴有低热起伏、盗汗、骨蒸、舌光红少津、脉细数无力等阴竭症状。由于其病变本质属虚，所以其动风之状多较轻缓，常见于外感热病或久病的后遗症期及老年病人。

The term refers to the pathological change due to the exhaustion of liver yin and kidney yin giving rise to sinews being deprived of nourishment and wind being stirred internally. Yin deficiency generating wind is often caused by yin-fluid insufficiency in the late stage of febrile diseases, yin consumption due to chronic diseases, or natural consumption of yin fluids in the liver and the kidney due to aging. Insufficiency makes yin fluids unable to nourish and moisten sinews and vessels, which produces internal wind. Clinically, it is manifested as limb wriggling and muscle twitching, accompanied with such symptoms of yin exhaustion as tidal low-grade fever, night sweat, bone steaming, red tongue with little coating and saliva, and thready rapid weak pulse. As this is a pathological change of deficiency in nature, its symptoms of stirring wind are mostly mild and moderate and commonly seen in elderly patients and patients with sequelae of externally-contracted febrile diseases or chronic illnesses.

【曾经译法】 /

【现行译法】 interior wind due to yin-deficiency; yin-asthenia producing wind; yin-deficiency generating wind

【标准译法】 Yin deficiency generates wind.

【翻译说明】 "阴虚"和"风"的译法都比较固定，译为 yin deficiency 和 wind，意思准确，并与中文术语对应。"生"译为 produce

或 generate。《新牛津英汉双解大词典》对 generate 的解释为 cause (something, especially an emotion or situation) to arise or come about, 可表示"造成，引起，导致"，较符合语境。

引例 Citations:

◎此阴虚生风，非指外感之邪也。（《本草述钩元》卷二十四）

（这个是阴虚生风，而并不是指外感邪气。）

It denotes yin deficiency generates wind rather than external contraction of pathogenic qi. (*Delving into the Description of Materia Medica*)

◎气虚生痰，阴虚生风，风邪挟痰走窜经隧，不能流利机关。（《陈莲舫医案集》）

（气虚而生痰，阴虚而生风，风邪兼夹痰浊走窜于经络，致使关节不滑利。）

Qi deficiency generates phlegm, and yin deficiency generates wind. Wind pathogen with phlegm runs through the meridians, resulting in stiff joints. (*Case Records of Chen Lianfang*)

◎肝胃阴虚，风动肢痿者，主通摄（熟地、牛膝、远志、杞子、石斛、钩藤。）（《类证治裁》卷五）

（肝胃阴液亏虚，动风而肢痿的，治疗应疏通收摄，药用熟地、牛膝、远志、杞子、石斛、钩藤。）

Cases of liver-and-stomach yin deficiency, in which wind is generated and limb atrophy occurs, could be treated with dredging and astringing therapies. Medicinal substances to be used include *shudi* (*Radix Rehmanniae Praeparata*, prepared rehmannia root), *niuxi* (*Radix Achyranthis Bidentatae*, two-toothed achyranthes root), *yuanzhi* (*Radix Polygalae*, thin-leaf milkwort root), *qizi* (*Fructus Lycii*, Chinese wolfberry fruit), *shihu* (*Caulis Dendrobii*, dendrobium stem), and *gouteng* (*Ramulus Uncariae Cum Uncis*, gambir plant). (*Categorized Patterns with Clear-cut Treatments*)

血虚生风

Blood Deficiency Generates Wind.

血液亏虚，筋脉失养，虚风内动的病理变化。血虚生风多因生血不足或失血过多，或久病耗伤营血，肝血不足，筋脉失养，或血不荣络所致。临床可见肢体麻木、筋肉跳动，甚或手足震颤或拘挛不伸等症状，并兼有血虚表现。其病变本质属虚，故动风之状也较轻缓。

The term refers to the pathological change due to blood deficiency giving rise to poor nourishment of sinews and internal stirring of deficient wind. It is often caused by insufficient blood production or massive blood loss. Another cause is insufficient liver blood failing to nourish the sinews due to the consumption and damage of nutrient blood caused by chronic diseases. The third reason is that blood fails to nourish collaterals. Clinically, it is manifested as limb numbness, sinew and muscle twitching, and even limb tremor and spasms, accompanied with symptoms of blood deficiency. As this pathological change is a deficiency pattern in nature, its symptoms of stirring wind are relatively mild and moderate.

【曾经译法】 Deficiency of blood may cause wind-syndrome; blood deficiency producing wind; Wind Syndrome due to Blood Deficiency

【现行译法】 interior wind due to blood-deficiency; blood-asthenia generating wind; blood-deficiency producing wind; blood deficiency producing wind; generation of endogenous wind due to blood deficiency; syndrome/pattern of blood deficiency with generation of wind; pattern/syndrome of blood deficiency engendering wind; blood deficiency producing wind; syndrome/pattern of blood deficiency producing wind

【标准译法】 Blood deficiency generates wind.

【翻译说明】 "血虚"和"风"的译法都比较固定，译为 blood deficiency

和 wind。"生"译为 cause, produce, generate 和 engender。依据《新牛津英汉双解大词典》,generate 可表示"造成,引起,导致",较符合语境。

引例 Citations:

◎若见惊搐等证,肝经血虚生风也,四物加天麻、钩藤钩。(《张氏医通》卷十一)

（若出现惊搐等症状,是肝经血虚而生风,治疗用四物汤加天麻、钩藤钩。）

If convulsive seizure or similar symptoms occur, it is because blood deficiency in the liver meridian generates wind. *Siwu* Decoction (Four Ingredients Decoction) plus *tianma* (*Rhizoma Gastrodiae*, tall gastrodis tuber) and *goutenggou* (*Ramulus Uncariae Cum Uncis*, gambir plant) should be used for treatment. (*Comprehensive Medicine by Doctor Zhang Lu*)

◎失血之人,血虚生风者,多逍遥散加川芎、青葙子、夏枯草治之。(《血证论》卷六)

（大出血的病人,血虚而生风的,多用逍遥散加川芎、青葙子、夏枯草治疗。）

For patients with massive blood loss and whose blood deficiency generates wind, *Xiaoyao* Powder (Free Wanderer Powder) should be used with *chuanxiong* (*Rhizoma Chuanxiong*, Sichuan lovage rhizome), *qingxiangzi* (*Semen Celosiae*, feather cockscomb seed), and *xiakucao* (*Spica Prunellae*, common self-heal fruit-spike). (*Treatise on Blood Syndromes*)

◎独活寄生汤,治产后血虚生风,手足抽掣,筋脉挛急,时发搐搦,半身不遂。(《世医得效方》)

（独活寄生汤，主治产后血虚生风，手足抽掣，筋脉挛急，常发
生肌肉抽动，半身不遂。）

Duhuo Jisheng Decoction (Pubescent Angelica and Mistletoe Decoction) is mainly used to treat postpartum symptoms of blood deficiency generating wind such as convulsion of hands and feet, sinew spasms and tension, frequent muscle twitching, and hemiplegia. (*Effective Formulas from Generations of Physicians*) rèjí shēng fēng

热极生风

Extreme Heat Generates Wind.

邪热炽盛，伤及营血，燔灼肝经，筋脉失养而挛急抽搐的病理变化。热极生风多由于邪热炽盛，煎灼津液，伤及营血，燔灼肝筋，使筋脉失其柔顺之性。临床可见痉厥、四肢抽搐、目睛上吊、角弓反张等症状，并伴有高热、神昏、谵语等症。其主要病机是邪热亢盛，属于实性病变，多见于外感热病的极期。

The term refers to the pathological change caused by intense pathogenic heat which damages nutrient blood, scorches the liver meridian, and deprives sinews of nourishment, leading to spasm, tension, and convulsion. Its pathogenesis is that intense pathogenic heat dries body fluids, damages nutrient blood, scorches the liver meridian, and causes sinews to become stiff and taut. Clinically, it is manifested as convulsive syncope, convulsion of the limbs, showing the whites of eyes, and opisthotonus, accompanied with high fever, loss of consciousness, delirious speech, etc. As its pathogenesis is attributable to the hyperactivity of heat pathogen, it is an excess pattern in nature, often seen at the fastigium of externally-contracted febrile diseases.

【曾经译法】 EXTREME HEAT BRINGING ABOUT WIND; extreme heat causing wind; Extreme Heat causes Wind; over-heat generating wind

【现行译法】 interior wind due to overabundance of pathogenic heat; extreme heat producing wind; excessive heat generating wind; intense heat generating wind; syndrome/pattern of extreme heat with generation of wind; extreme heat engendering wind

【标准译法】 Extreme heat generates wind.

【翻译说明】 "极"被译为 extreme, over-, overabundance, excessive 和 intense，其中，extreme 的意思与术语原文最为对应，可以与

heat（热）搭配，在现有译文中使用频率也最高，推广性也最好。"生"译为 bring about, cause, generate, produce 或 engender。其中，generate 可表示"产生"或"造成，引起，导致"，故采用。

引例 Citations:

◎或热极生风而热燥郁，舌强口噤，筋惕肉瞤。（《黄帝素问宣明论方》卷三）

（或者热极生风，燥热内郁，舌强口噤，筋肉不自主地惕然瘛动。）

Or extreme heat generates wind, i.e., internal constraint of dryness-heat causes stiff tongue, lockjaw, and muscle twitching. (*Profound Formulas Inspired by the Yellow Emperor's Plain Conversation*)

◎大抵小儿为病，多因热极生风，风生惊，故有热即当清之。（《简明医彀》卷六）

（大部分小儿疾病，多因为热极生风，因风而惊，因此有热应立即清热。）

Most pediatric diseases are caused by extreme heat generating wind, which leads to infantile convulsion, so heat should be cleared as soon as it appears. (*Concise Medical Guidelines*)

◎此法治热极生风之证，故用连翘、竹叶以清其热。（《时病论》卷四）

（这一方法治疗热极生风的病证，所以用连翘、竹叶以清除热邪。）

This therapy is used to treat the pattern of extreme heat generating wind, so *lianqiao* (*Fructus Forsythiae*, weeping forsythia capsule) and *zhuye* (*Folium Phyllostachydis Henonis*, henon bamboo leaf) are used to clear the heat. (*Treatise on Seasonal Diseases*) xuèzào shēng fēng

血燥生风

Blood Dryness Generates Wind.

血虚津亏，失润化燥，肌肤失于濡养而致干燥瘙痒及脱屑的病理变化。血燥生风多因久病耗伤精血，或年老精亏血少，或长期饮食失宜，营血生成不足，或瘀血内结，新血化生障碍，从而导致津枯血少，肌肤失于濡养而化风。临床以皮肤干燥或肌肤甲错、皮肤瘙痒、脱屑为特征。

The term refers to the pathological change manifested as dry and itchy skin as well as desquamation caused by the deficiency of blood and fluids which fail to moisten and nourish the muscles and skin. Blood dryness generating endogenous wind is often caused by consumption of essence and blood due to chronic diseases, deficiency of essence and blood due to senility, insufficiency of blood generation due to long-term improper diet, or malfunction of blood generation due to accumulation of static blood, leading to depletion of fluids and blood which brings failure to moisten and nourish the muscles and skin and transforming into wind. Clinically, it is marked by dry or scaly skin, itching, and skin desquamation.

【曾经译法】blood-dryness producing endogenous wind

【现行译法】blood dryness generating/producing wind; Dryness in blood generates internal wind; blood dryness causing wind; blood dryness producing wind

【标准译法】Blood dryness generates wind.

【翻译说明】"生"被译为 produce, generate 或 cause，其中，generate 可表示"产生"或"造成，引起，导致"，故采用。

引例 Citations:

◎妇人赤白游风，属肝经怒火，血燥生风。(《妇人大全良方》卷二十四)

　　(妇女得了赤白游风，是因为肝经怒火，血燥生风。)

Urticaria in women is caused by the anger-fire in the liver meridian and the endogenous wind due to blood dryness. (*Complete Effective Prescriptions for Women's Diseases*)

◎若肌肤干燥，瘦削痒痛，搔破出血，或无血而起白屑，此乃血燥生风，风郁化热。(《外证医案汇编》卷四)

　　(如果皮肤干燥，瘦削痒痛，搔破出血，或者不出血而起白皮屑，
　　这是由于血燥生风，风郁化热所致。)

Dry skin, thinness, itching, pain, bleeding from scratches, or white scurf from scratches without bleeding are caused by endogenous wind due to blood dryness and the heat resulting from constrained wind. (*Collection of Case Records in External Patterns*)

◎凡证属肝经血燥生风者，但宜滋肾水生肝血，则火自息，风自定，痒自止。(《景岳全书》卷三十四)

　　(凡证属于肝经血燥生风的患者，治疗只需滋肾水生肝血，这样
　　火就自然会熄灭，风就自然会安定，瘙痒自然会停止。)

Patients with blood dryness generating wind in the liver meridian should be treated by nourishing kidney water and engendering liver blood, which quenches the fire and extinguishes the wind to stop itching. (*Jingyue's Complete Works*) tǔyōng mùyù

土壅木郁

Earth Stagnation Causes Wood Depression.

　　脾气壅滞，升降失常，导致肝失疏泄的病理变化。又称为土反侮木、脾湿肝郁等。依据脏腑五行归属关系，脾属土，肝属木。由于饮食不节，损伤脾胃，使脾失健运，湿浊内生，困于脾土，气滞中焦，升降失司，导致肝之疏泄失职，临床表现先有湿困脾土的纳呆、腹胀、食少、便溏、苔腻等症状，继之再出现两胁胀痛、精神抑郁等肝郁的表现。若湿热困脾，影响肝胆疏泄，胆汁上溢外泛，可见口苦、黄疸等症状。

The term refers to the pathological change in which the stagnation of spleen qi and its disorder of ascending and descending cause the failure of the liver to govern the free flow of qi. It is also known as liver depression due to spleen dampness, or earth counter-restricting wood as the spleen pertains to earth and the liver pertains to wood according to the five-element theory. Improper diet impairs the spleen and the stomach, causing the failure of the spleen to transport and the occurrence of internal dampness. The spleen earth is thus encumbered, incurring qi stagnation in the middle energizer and its disorder of ascending and descending, making the liver unable to govern the free flow of qi. Clinically, it is marked by poor digestion, abdominal distention, poor appetite, loose stools, and greasy tongue coating due to dampness encumbering the spleen. Subsequent symptoms include hypochondriac distending pain and mental depression caused by liver-qi stagnation. Bitter taste in mouth and jaundice may occur if damp-heat encumbers the spleen to affect the liver in governing the free flow of qi, causing the counterflow and overflow of bile.

【曾经译法】 /

【现行译法】 earth stagnation and wood depression

【标准译法】 Earth stagnation causes wood depression.

【翻译说明】 脾土主运化，为气之枢纽。"壅"为"壅滞、堵塞"之意，译为 stagnation。"郁"为"抑郁"之意，译为 depression，符合脾气壅滞，气机升降失常，导致肝郁的意思。

引例 Citations:

◎胃病者，腹䐜胀，胃脘当心而痛，上支两胁（胁为肝部，土反侮木）。（《素问灵枢类纂约注》卷中）

（胃病患者，腹部胀满，胃脘靠近心口的部位疼痛，并向上顶着两胁部。两胁是肝经循行的部位，这是由于脾气壅滞，导致肝失疏泄。）

Patients with stomach disorders present symptoms such as abdominal distension, and pain in the upper stomach near the precordium, with obstructive feeling in the hypochondriac region where the liver meridian travels. They are manifestations of spleen-qi stagnation causing the failure of the liver to govern the free flow of qi. (*Classified Compilation and Concise Annotation of "Plain Conversation" and "Spiritual Pivot"*)

◎脾主肉，形有余则脾湿肝郁，腹胀泾溲不利。（《素问悬解》卷八）

（脾脏主宰肌肉，形体有余则湿困脾土，肝失疏泄，表现为腹胀满，大小便不利。）

The spleen governs muscles, and thus excess of the body indicates spleen dampness encumbers the liver and the liver fails to govern the free flow of qi, presenting symptoms of abdominal distension and inhibited urination and defecation. (*Explanation of Unresolved Issues in "Plain Conversation"*)

◎痰气交阻，土滞木郁，肝木从而不平。(《张聿青医案》)

　　(痰气交互阻滞，脾气壅滞，肝气郁结，导致肝的功能失调。)

Binding of phlegm and qi, causes stagnation of spleen qi and depression of liver qi, giving rise to liver dysfunction. (*Case Records of Zhang Yuqing*) tǔ bù zhìshuǐ

土不制水

Earth Fails to Control Water.

脾土虚弱不能运化、制约水湿，致湿浊停滞，泛滥为患的病理变化。依据脏腑五行归属关系，脾属土，肾主水。在正常情况下，脾土制约水液，使其正常运化，不使泛滥成病。若脾土虚弱，不能制约水湿，则可泛滥为患，出现水肿、痰饮等症。

The term refers to the pathological change characterized by stagnation and overflow of damp-turbidity due to weak spleen earth failing to transport, transform and control fluids and dampness. According to the five-element theory, the spleen pertains to earth and the kidney pertains to water. Normally spleen earth controls water to achieve proper transportation and transformation, preventing pathological overflow. However, when spleen earth is weak and fails to control water, overflow problems may occur and symptoms such as edema and phlegm-rheum can be found.

【曾经译法】 INHIBITION OF EARTH TO TRANSPORT WATER; Earth fails to control water; Earth fails to restrain water; Spleen fails to restrict Water (Kidney)

【现行译法】 Earth fails to restrict water; earth failing to control water; failure of earth to restrain water; spleen failing to restrain kidney; earth (spleen) failing to control water (kidney)

【标准译法】 Earth fails to control water.

【翻译说明】 "制"被译为 inhibit, restrict, control 或 restrain。其中，control 侧重指对事物的控制，更能体现脾土对水湿的管制之意。"土不制水"中的"不"理解为"不能够"，译为 fail 较恰当。

引例 Citations:

◎今真火气亏，不能滋养真土，故土不制水，水液妄行，三焦不泻，气脉闭塞，枢机不通，喘息奔急，水气盈溢，渗透经络，皮肤溢满，足胫尤甚，两目下肿。(《三因极一病证方论》卷十四)

（现在肾阳亏虚，不能温煦脾阳，所以脾土虚弱，不能制约水湿，使水液妄行，三焦水道不畅，气脉闭塞，人体气机不通，所以喘息奔急；水气盈溢，渗透经络，皮肤水肿，足胫尤其明显，两目下肿。）

Deficient kidney yang is unable to warm spleen yang, causing the weakness of spleen earth and its failure to control water. Thus, there may occur frenetic flowing of water, obstruction in the waterway of triple energizer, and blocking of qi in meridians. When qi movement in the human body is impaired, panting consequently occurs; when uncontrolled water permeates the meridians and collaterals, edema occurs, especially in the legs, feet, and under the eyes. (*Discussion of Pathology Based on Triple Etiology Doctrine*)

◎往往脾气既衰，元气耗散，土不制水，故水溢不收。(《杨氏家藏方》)

（往往脾气已经虚衰，元气耗散，脾土虚弱，不能制约水湿，所以水液泛滥为患。）

Usually with declined spleen qi and exhausted original qi, spleen earth is too weak to control water so that water overflow problems occur. (*Reserved Formulas of Yang's Family*)

◎夫痰即水也，其本在肾，其标在脾……在脾者，以食饮不化，土不制水也。(《景岳全书·杂证谟》)

（痰就是由水转化的，其产生的根本在肾，其标在脾……痰在脾而生者，是由于脾失健运，食饮不化，不能制约水湿。）

Phlegm is transformed from water, originating from the kidney and produced by the spleen… That phlegm is produced by the spleen is due to the failure of the spleen to transport and transform food and drinks as well as to control water and dampness. (*Jingyue's Complete Works*) mùhuǒ xíng jīn

木火刑金

Wood Fire Impairs Metal.

肝火炽盛，上逆犯肺，肺失清肃的病理变化。又称肝火犯肺。依据脏腑五行归属关系，肝属木，肺属金。在生理上，肝气升发，肺气肃降，两者相互制约，相反相成，不使太过或不及。若肝气郁结，气郁化火，灼伤肺络，肺失清肃，临床可见心烦易怒、胸胁疼痛、口苦、目赤、咳逆、咯血等症状。

The term refers to the pathological change caused by the ascending counterflow of intense liver fire impairing the lung to purify qi. It is also known as liver fire invading the lung. According to the five-element theory, the liver pertains to wood and the lung pertains to metal; hence the name. Physiologically, liver qi ascends, while lung qi descends. They are opposite but complementary, restricting each other to prevent excess or insufficiency. If liver qi is constrained, qi depression can transform into fire, and fire may scorch the lung collaterals and impair the lung to purify qi. Hence, clinical symptoms may occur including vexation, irritability, chest and hypochondriac pain, bitter taste in mouth, redness of eyes, cough, dyspnea, and hemoptysis.

【曾经译法】 WOOD FIRE DAMAGING METAL; Wood-fire impairs metal; Wood-Fire Burns Metal

【现行译法】 wood-fire impairing metal; wood fire tormenting metal; wood (liver) fire tormenting metal (lung)

【标准译法】 Wood fire impairs metal.

【翻译说明】 "刑"被译为 damage, impair, burn 或 torment, 其中, impair 表示对某物造成伤害或者使某物变得更糟糕，其意思符合肝火伤及肺络，从而导致各种症状的病理基础。

引例 Citations:

◎嗽血失音，且形瘦面赤，从木火刑金治。(《扫叶庄一瓢老人医案》卷一)

（咳血失音，并且形体消瘦、面红，按木火刑金治疗。）

Cough with blood, loss of voice, emaciation, and redness of face are the symptoms of wood fire impairing metal and should be treated accordingly. (*Case Records of Elderly Yipiao in Saoye House*)

◎咳嗽者，木火刑金也，止嗽散加柴胡、枳壳、赤芍主之。(《笔花医镜》卷二)

（咳嗽，属木火刑金证的，用止嗽散加柴胡、枳壳、赤芍治疗。）

Cough due to wood fire impairing metal should be treated with *Zhisou* Powder (Cough-stopping Powder) plus *chaihu* (*Radix Bupleuri*, Chinese thorowax root), *zhiqiao* (*Fructus Aurantii*, orange fruit), and *chishao* (*Radix Paeoniae Rubra*, peony root). (*Bihua's Medical Works*)

◎木火刑金，咳呛不止，甚则呕恶，治以清润肝肺为主。(《繫山草堂医案》卷上)

（木火刑金所致的呛咳不止，甚则呕恶，治疗以清肝润肺为主。）

Persistent coughing and chocking, even vomiting and nausea, caused by wood fire impairing metal should be treated mainly by clearing the liver and moistening the lung. (*Case Records of Ganshan Cottage*)

子盗母气

Child Organ Affects Mother Organ.

用五行相生母子关系，说明五脏之间子脏虚损累及母脏的病机传变。如脾土为母，肺金为子，肺气虚弱，肺病及脾，子盗母气，致脾气不运，气化乏源，故见脘痞、神疲乏力、面白无华、消瘦等症状。又如肝与心为母子之脏，若心血不足引起肝血亏虚，终致心肝血虚等。

The term refers to the pathogenesis of deficient child organ affecting mother organ in accordance with the generation among the five elements (i.e., zang-organs). For instance, spleen earth is the mother organ and lung metal is the child organ. The deficiency of lung qi can affect the spleen, i.e., child organ affects mother organ, thus impairing the transportation of spleen qi and causing the lack of source in transforming qi. Clinically, it is marked by gastric stuffiness, fatigue, pale and lusterless complexion, emaciation, etc. Another example concerns the mother-child relationship between the liver and the heart. Insufficiency of heart blood will give rise to deficiency of liver blood, resulting in heart-liver blood deficiency.

【曾经译法】 Illness of a child-organ may involve its mother organ; illness of the child stealing the mother-qi

【现行译法】 Illness of the child organ may involve the mother organ; child-organ disease affecting the mother-organ; Child-organ steals qi from its mother-organ; disorder of child-organ affecting mother-organ

【标准译法】 Child organ affects mother organ.

【翻译说明】 "子盗母气"中的"子"和"母"应理解为"子脏"和"母脏"，用 child 和 mother 表示两者之间的关系。将"盗"意译为 affect 较好，因为 steal 有将他物据为己有的含义，与子脏伤及母脏的语义不符。省去（child-organ）illness 是为了保持术语的简洁性。"气"在此处并非表示气之实体，而是指代脏腑功能，故省略不译。

引例 Citations:

◎夜不寐者，由子盗母气，心虚而神不安也。(《石山医案》卷下)

（失眠，是由于子盗母气，心气虚而精神不安。）

Insomnia occurs due to heart-qi deficiency caused by child organ affecting mother organ which gives rise to restlessness of the spirit and mind. (*Shishan's Case Records*)

◎若见白色，则子盗母气，虚邪也。(《望诊遵经》)

（如果面色白，是由于子盗母气，邪气乘虚而入。）

Pale complexion is the result of invasion by pathogenic qi when healthy qi is weakened due to child organ affecting mother organ. (*Principles Followed in Inspection Diagnosis*)

◎由于肾虚，火烁金伤，子盗母气，声哑喉疼，咳吐粉红脓血。(《问斋医案》卷三)

（由于肾阴虚，虚火灼伤肺金，子盗母气，就出现声音嘶哑，咽喉疼痛，咳吐粉红脓血等症。）

Symptoms such as hoarse voice, sore throat, and cough with pink pus or blood occur due to kidney-yin deficiency which causes deficiency fire scorching lung metal, a pattern of child organ affecting mother organ. (*Wenzhai's Case Records*) mǔbìng jí zǐ

母病及子

Mother Organ Affects Child Organ.

用五行相生母子关系，说明五脏之间由于母脏病变累及子脏的病机传变。如肾属水，肝属木，水能生木，故肾为母脏，肝为子脏。肾病波及于肝，即属母病及子。临床上多表现为肾阴不足不能滋养肝木，导致肝阴虚而阴不制阳，出现肝阳上亢证。

The term refers to the pathogenesis of mother organ affecting child organ in accordance with the generation among the five elements (i.e., zang-organs). For instance, the kidney pertains to water and the liver pertains to wood, and water generates wood; therefore, the kidney is the mother organ and the liver is the child organ. If a kidney disease affects the liver, it is described as mother organ affecting child organ. Clinically, it is marked by liver-yang hyperactivity—a result of kidney yin being too deficient to nourish liver wood, causing liver-yin deficiency, and thus making yin fail to restrict yang.

【曾经译法】 A MATERNAL DISEASE AFFECTING ITS OFFSPRING; Illness of a mother-organ may involve its child organ; diseased mother affecting the child; Illness of the mother organ affects the child one

【现行译法】 disorders of the mother organ affecting the child organ; disorder of the mother-organ involving the child-organ; disorder of the mother-organ affecting its child-organ; illness of mother viscera affecting the child one; disorder of mother-organ affecting child-organ

【标准译法】 Mother organ affects child organ.

【翻译说明】 "母病及子"中的"母"和"子"应理解为"母脏"和"子脏"，用 mother 和 child 表示两者之间的关系。"及"意为"累及"，说明母脏的病变会累及子脏，对子脏产生影响，故用 affect。

引例 Citations:

◎肺属金，金之母土也，胃土湿热未清，上焦肺部焉得不受其熏蒸，所谓母病及子也。(《柳选四家医案》卷七)

（肺在五行属金，金的母为土也，胃土湿热未清，必然熏蒸上焦肺部，这就是母病及子。）

According to the five-element theory, the lung pertains to metal whose mother is earth. If the damp-heat in the stomach earth remains uncleared, it is bound to steam the lung in the upper energizer. This exemplifies the pattern of mother organ affecting child organ. (*Case Records of Four Doctors Selected by Liu Baozhi*)

◎更有母病及子者，如金病而移于肾是也。(《医理真传》卷一)

（更有母病及子的，例如肺病转移到肾。）

There is a pattern of mother organ affecting child organ. For example, lung disease can cause kidney disorders. (*True Transmission of Medical Principles*)

◎脉浮为虚，弦者母病及子，肾传肝也。(《素问释义》卷十)

（脉浮为虚证，脉弦为母病及子，由肾传到肝。）

Floating pulse indicates deficiency pattern, while wiry pulse suggests mother organ affecting child organ, which is the result of a kidney illness affecting the liver. (*Interpretation of Plain Conversation*) jīnshí bù míng

金实不鸣

A Solid Bell Cannot Ring.

肺气实所致声哑，甚或失音的病理变化。喉为肺之门户，是清浊之气出入之要道，发音的主要器官。发音是肺气鼓动喉之声带而发出，故为肺所主。生理情况下，肺气宣畅，肺阴充足，则呼吸通利，声音宏亮清晰。病理情况下，若风寒、风热犯肺，可使肺气失宣，出现声音嘶哑或失音、喉痒、喉痛等症。由于肺在五行属金，故称为"金实不鸣"。

The term refers to the pathological change manifested as hoarse voice or even aphonia due to excess lung qi. The larynx is the gateway to the lung, the thoroughfare for the exiting and entering path of clear and turbid qi, and the main vocal organ. Lung qi causes the vocal cords in the larynx to vibrate and produce sound, and thus the lung governs sound. Physiologically, free and smooth flow of lung qi and sufficient lung yin jointly contribute to unobstructed breathing as well as loud and clear voice. Pathologically, if the lung is attacked by wind-cold or wind-heat, lung qi is unable to disperse normally, and symptoms such as hoarse voice, aphonia, itchy throat, and throat pain can occur. Since the lung pertains to metal in accordance with the five-element theory, the pathological change is described as the pattern that "a solid bell cannot ring."

【曾经译法】 DYSPHONIA DUE TO EXCESSIVE METAL; solid bell cannot be sounded; A stuffed bell does not ring

【现行译法】 A solid bell cannot ring; A solid bell cannot ring (hoarseness or dysphonia due to sthenia lung syndrome); hoarseness due to attack by external pathogenic factors; obstructed lung not functioning normally; muffled metal failing to sound

【标准译法】 A solid bell cannot ring.

【翻译说明】 古人用钟鸣很好地比喻了喉发声，其相通之处在于钟的材

158

质为金属，而以喉为门户的肺在五行中属金。此处采用直译，描述大钟的空腔因变实而无法鸣响，能够更直观地反映失音和肺实之间的关系。"实"一词的翻译选取 solid 而非 muffled，是由于肺的实证往往为邪实壅塞，声音本身难以产生，而非被外物蒙住而无法传声，其症结在于肺（钟）本身，而非传导途径。

引例 Citations:

◎失音大都不越于肺，然须以暴病得之，为邪郁气逆，久病得之，为津枯血槁……昔人所谓金实不鸣，金破亦不鸣也。（《张氏医通》卷四）

（失音大多和肺关系密切，但必须是急性病引起的，多是邪气郁结、气机上逆；慢性病引起的，多因津血亏虚……古人所谓的金实不鸣，金破也不鸣。）

In most cases, aphonia indicates lung diseases. It must be caused by acute illnesses as a result of binding constraint of pathogenic qi and ascending counterflow of qi, or by chronic illnesses as a result of exhaustion of fluids and blood… This is described as the pattern that a solid bell cannot ring or a broken bell cannot ring. (*Comprehensive Medicine by Doctor Zhang Lu*)

◎有嗽而声哑者，盖金实不鸣，金破亦不鸣。实则清之，破则补之，皆治肺之事也。（《医贯》卷四）

（咳嗽并且声音嘶哑的患者，大概是金实不鸣，或金破不鸣。对于金实不鸣者采用清泻法治疗，金破不鸣者采用补益法治疗，都是从肺论治。）

Coughing and hoarse voice are often the manifestations of the pattern that a solid bell cannot ring or a broken bell cannot ring. Patients with "a solid bell" should be treated with clearing and purging method, while those with "a broken bell" should be treated with supplementing therapy. The lung is the target for treatment in both cases. (*Key Link of Medicine*)

◎咳而失音，有新久虚实之异。新者多实，痰火闭郁，所谓金实不鸣也。久者多虚，肺损气脱，所谓金破亦不鸣也。(《金匮翼》卷七)

　　(咳嗽而失音，有新久虚实的差别。新病者多为实证，因痰火闭郁所致，所谓金实不鸣。久病者多虚证，常因肺气虚脱所致，所谓金破不鸣。)

Aphonia caused by coughing can be classified into four types: recently acquired, long-standing, deficiency, and excess. The recently acquired disorder often falls into the excess type, characterized by phlegm-fire obstruction and constraint described as the pattern that a solid bell cannot ring. The long-standing one often falls into the deficiency type, characterized by lung impairment and qi collapse described as the pattern that a broken bell cannot ring. (*Supplements for the Understanding of "Essential Prescriptions of the Golden Cabinet"*) jīnpò bù míng

金破不鸣

A Broken Bell Cannot Ring.

肺气阴虚损，津亏失润而声哑，甚或失音的病理变化。肺在五行属金，若肺气耗伤，肺阴不足，虚火内灼，可见音声低微，声音嘶哑或失音，或喉部干涩微痛等症，故称为"金破不鸣"。

The term refers to the pathological change manifested as hoarse voice or even aphonia due to fluid consumption and the lack of moistening as a result of impairment and deficiency of lung qi and lung yin. According to the five-element theory, the lung pertains to metal. If lung qi is impaired and lung yin is insufficient, deficiency fire will scorch internally, causing symptoms such as faint voice, hoarseness or even aphonia, or dry and slightly painful throat, which is described as the pattern that "a broken bell cannot ring."

【曾经译法】 dysphonia due to broken metal; Broken bell-metal cannot ring; A broken bell does not ring

【现行译法】 A broken gong does not sound; A broken bell does not sound (aphonia due to sthenia of pulmonary qi; sudden aphonia); hoarseness due to lung dysfunction; damaged lung not functioning normally; broken metal failing to sound

【标准译法】 A broken bell cannot ring.

【翻译说明】 古人用钟鸣很好地比喻了喉发声，其相通之处在于钟的材质为金属，而以喉为门户的肺在五行中属金。此处采用直译，描述大钟因破损而无法鸣响，能够更直观地反映失音和肺虚之间的关系。

引例 Citations:

◎有嗽而声哑者，盖金实不鸣，痰火郁于中也；金破亦不鸣，肺气伤于内也。(《疡医大全》卷十七)

（有咳嗽而声音嘶哑的，大概属金实不鸣，痰火郁于肺所致；也有属于金破不鸣，肺气内伤所致。）

Hoarse voice due to coughing is possibly caused by the constraint of phlegm-fire in the lung, which is described as the pattern that a solid bell cannot ring, or by the impairment of lung qi, which is described as the pattern that a broken bell cannot ring. (*A Complete Collection of Sore and Wound Treatment*)

◎痨伤咳嗽主乎内也，二者不治，至于咳嗽失音，是金破不鸣矣。(《医学三字经》卷一)

（痨伤、咳嗽病生于内，二者没有及时治疗，导致咳嗽失音，这是金破不鸣。）

Impairment from consumptive disease and cough caused by endogenous pathogens, if not treated in time, will result in aphonia. This falls into the pattern that a broken bell cannot ring. (*Three-character Medical Verses*)

四气调神

Regulating Life Activities According to Seasonal Changes

顺应四时气候、物候变化，调养人体神志活动。由于四时阴阳为万物之根本，万物皆生于春，长于夏，收于秋，藏于冬，人亦应之。故养生也要顺应四时气候、物候的变化，使人体生命活动与自然界四时保持协调一致。具体而言，在生活起居方面，春夏宜晚卧早起，多到室外散步，舒展形体，适当从事户外活动，目的在于促进阳气的生发、盛长、宣泄；秋冬则要顺应自然界肃杀、闭藏的变化，尽量早睡，适当减少运动，避免外寒侵袭，目的在于收敛、固藏阳气。从精神调摄而言，春夏宜放松，精神欢快，使神气舒畅；秋冬宜神志淡静，精神内敛，使神气内藏。

The term refers to the regulation of life activities in accordance with the climatic and phenological changes in the four seasons. Through the four seasons, the change of yin and yang is the root of life, characterized by sprouting in spring, growing in summer, harvesting in autumn, and storing in winter, a rule that human beings should comply with. Therefore, health preservation practice should be in concert with the climatic and phenological changes in the four seasons in order to maintain harmony between human life activities and natural seasonal changes. Specifically, in terms of everyday life, one should go to bed late and get up early in spring and summer months. To promote the growing, thriving, and dispersing of yang qi, one should also take strolls, stretch body, and moderately take part in outdoor activities. In autumn and winter time, to comply with the characteristics of elimination, concealment, and storage in nature, one should go to bed early, reduce activities proportionally, and avoid attack by external cold for the sake of astringing and storing yang qi. In terms of regulating spirit, it is preferable to relax and stay joyful in spring and summer in order to keep the smooth flow of qi, while it is better to keep peaceful and calm and maintain a restrained spirit in autumn and winter in order to store qi and spirit.

【曾经译法】regulating life activities according to natural changes in four seasons

【现行译法】regulating life activities according to seasonal changes

【标准译法】regulating life activities according to seasonal changes

【翻译说明】"四气"指四季呈现的各种气候与物候变化，选用 seasonal changes 而非 natural changes in four seasons，是为强调气候、物候因季节造成的变化，而不仅仅是四季间发生的变化。"神"指神志等生命活动，故译为 life activities。

引例 Citations:

◎以四气调神，以五运明化，相生有子母之道，相克有夫妇之义。(《宋徽宗圣济经》卷七)

（按照四时气候、物候变化，调养人体神志活动；依据五运来推求气候变化，相生有类似于母子的规律，相克有类似于夫妇的规律。）

Life activities should be regulated according to seasonal changes. Climate change can be deduced according to the theory of five circuits. The generation cycle resembles the relationship between mother and child; the restriction cycle, husband and wife. (*Classic of Holy Benevolence by Emperor Huizong of the Song Dynasty*)

◎张氏用药，依准四时阴阳升降而增损之，正《内经》四气调神之义。(《医学纲目》卷三)

（张氏用药，依据四时阴阳升降变化而增减药物，符合《内经》四气调神的意义。）

In Zhang's customary prescription, the addition and subtraction of medicinals are in accordance with the ascending or descending of yin and yang in the four seasons, which corresponds with the rule of "regulating life activities according to seasonal changes" in *Yellow Emperor's Internal Canon of Medicine*. (*Compendium of Chinese Medicine*)

◎四气调神，乃圣人未病之治，未乱之防也。(《成方切用》卷末)

（按照四时气候、物候变化，调养人体神志活动，正是古代圣人治未病，防未乱的关键。）

Regulating life activities according to seasonal changes is the key to preventing diseases and disorders by ancient Chinese sages. (*Effective Use of Established Formulas*) tiándàn xūwú

恬惔虚无

Placidity and Nothingness

　　心境清静淡泊，无欲无求。中医学非常重视人的情志活动与身体健康的关系，认为人的情志活动的产生，是以人体内脏及内脏所化生的精微物质为基础，而精神情志活动又可以反作用于人体。因此，调摄精神，保养正气，就成为中医学养生防病的一个重要环节。而调神摄生，首在静养；静养之要，重在节欲，即要求人们做到对一切声名物欲应有所节制，达到虚怀若谷、淡泊名利、超然脱俗的精神境界，以避免不良情绪的产生，如此心静神藏，才能使人体脏腑气血和调，气机调畅，阴平阳秘，形神和谐，而健康长寿。

The term means that one is calm and serene in mind, free from all desires and wants. Traditional Chinese medicine (TCM) emphasizes the relationship between emotional activities and physical wellbeing, and considers the internal organs and the refined essence transformed by them are the basis for the generation of emotions which, in turn, can have an effect on the human body. Therefore, it is important to cultivate spiritual health and maintain healthy qi in terms of health preservation and disease prevention in TCM. For spirit regulation, the top priority is to cultivate inner peace, abstaining from excessive desires. In other words, one should refrain from wants and desires, taking a humble and compatible attitude, being indifferent to fame or wealth, and being detached and refined to avoid experiencing negative emotions. In so doing, one can maintain a tranquil mind and have the spirit stored so that zang-fu organs as well as qi and blood can be regulated, free flow of qi can be attained, yin and yang can remain stable and compact, and body-spirit harmony can be achieved. Thus, one enjoys health and longevity.

【曾经译法】/

【现行译法】calm and empty of cares and desires; tranquilized mind; indifferent to fame or gain; keep the mind pure and free from any avarice

【标准译法】placidity and nothingness

【翻译说明】"恬惔虚无"指心情清静安闲而没有杂念。译词 placidity 可表示"平静；平和"；nothingness 表示"虚无；不存在"。

引例 Citations:

◎恬惔虚无，真气从之，精神内守，病安从来？（《素问·上古天真论》）

（思想上清静淡泊，无欲无求，体内正气就会和顺不乱；精神守持于内而不耗散，那么疾病怎么会发生呢？）

Keep placidity and nothingness (free from all desires and wants), and healthy qi in the body will be in harmony, spirit will remain inside. If so, how can diseases occur? (*Plain Conversation*)

◎是以圣人为无为之事，乐恬惔之能，从欲快志于虚无之守，故寿命无穷，与天地终。（《素问·阴阳应象大论》）

（因此，圣人做的是顺应自然的事情，喜欢的是清静淡泊的生活状态，在无欲无求的境地自感适意、心情愉快，所以能够长生不老，跟天地一同结束生命。）

Thus, the sages never do anything against nature. They lead a placid life, free from all desires and wants, and feel at ease and happy. That is why they enjoy a natural life span. (*Plain Conversation*)

◎恬惔虚无，静也。法道清净，精气内持，故其气从，邪不能为害。（《黄帝内经素问》王冰注）

（恬惔虚无，即清静。效法"道"的清静，精气内守，顺从不乱，则邪气不能伤害人体。）

Placidity and nothingness refer to peace and quiet. Following the principle of peace and quiet in "Taoism," one can keep essential qi in the interior orderly and ward off pathogenic qi. (*Plain Conversation* in *Yellow Emperor's Internal Canon of Medicine* Annotated by Wang Bing)

知止不殆

Nothing Can Harm Who Stops in Time.

懂得适可而止，就不会带来危险。中医学非常重视人的情志与健康的关系，认为七情太过可直接伤及脏腑，引起气机紊乱而发病。而要避免不良情绪的产生，关键的一环是降低人的需要，知足、知止，以减少人的需求与客观事物之间的矛盾。如果过分地贪求种种声名物欲，所欲不遂就会产生忧郁、失望、悲伤、苦闷、恼怒等不良情绪，从而扰乱清静之神，导致气机紊乱而发病；只有少私寡欲，心静神藏，才可使脏腑气血和调，气机调畅，抗病力强，有利于延年益寿。

The term means the person who knows when to stop will not invite danger. Traditional Chinese medicine emphasizes the relationship between emotions and health, believing that the excess of seven emotions can bring direct harm to the zang-fu organs, causing qi-movement disorder and subsequent diseases. To prevent negative emotions, it is very important for people to reduce desires and understand what is enough and when to stop to reduce conflict between needs and reality. If a person has excessive wants and needs, he/she is likely to experience depression, disappointment, sadness, anguish, and anger when his/her desires are not met, resulting in a disturbance of spirit, disorder of qi movement, and subsequent diseases. Only with least desires, peace of mind, and well-stored spirit can one achieve qi-blood harmony in the zang-fu organs, free flow of qi, strong immunity, and longevity.

【曾经译法】/

【现行译法】/

【标准译法】Nothing can harm who stops in time.

【翻译说明】"知止不殆"可理解为"懂得适可而止，就不会带来危险"，直译为 The person who knows when to stop will not invite danger。

本词条参考 Arthur Waley 的译文，译为 Nothing can harm who stops in time。

引例 Citations:

◎名与身孰亲？身与货孰多？得与亡孰病？甚爱必大费，多藏必厚亡。故知足不辱，知止不殆，可以长久。（《老子》四十四章）

（声名和生命比起来哪一样亲切？生命和货利比起来哪一样贵重？得到名利和丧失生命哪一样为害？过分的爱名就必定要付出重大的耗费，过多的藏货就必定会招致惨重的损失。所以知道满足就不会受到屈辱，知道适可而止就不会带来危险，这样才可以保持长久。）

Fame or life, which is dearer? Life or wealth, which is more valuable? Between fame, wealth, and losing life, which is worse? Excessive love of fame costs greatly, and excessive hoard of goods invites catastrophic loss. Therefore, a person who is content with what he has will not be disgraced, and nothing can harm who stops in time. He is forever safe and secure. (*Laozi*)

◎高忘其贵，下安其分，两无相慕，知止不殆也。（《医经原旨·摄生第一》）

（地位高者忘记他的高贵，地位低下者安于本分，二者不相互羡慕，所谓懂得适可而止，就不会带来危险。）

One with higher status chooses to forget his privilege, while one with lower status is content with what he is. Neither is envious, and nothing can harm who stops in time. (*Original Decrees of Medicine*)

法于阴阳

Abiding by the Principle of Yin and Yang

养生要遵循自然界阴阳变化的规律。《黄帝内经》认为人的生命活动受自然界四时阴阳变化的影响与制约，因此养生必须顺应天地阴阳的变化，以调节人体的功能，增强对外界变化的适应能力，同时可以避免四时不正之气的侵袭。这一观点也成为后世养生保健的重要指导思想，历代养生专著无不把顺应自然界四时阴阳变化作为养生的重要内容。

Health preservation should be carried out in accordance with the principle of yin and yang in nature. According to *Yellow Emperor's Internal Canon of Medicine*, human life activities can be affected and restrained by climatic and phenological changes in the four seasons. Therefore, health should be preserved in accordance with the changes of yin and yang in nature to regulate physical functions, improve adaptability to environmental changes, and ward off pathogenic qi in the four seasons. The idea has since become an important guideline for health preservation and healthcare in later generations, and classics have never failed to include it throughout history.

【曾经译法】 according to Yin-Yang law

【现行译法】 abiding by law of yin and yang; following the rule of yin and yang

【标准译法】 abiding by the principle of yin and yang

【翻译说明】 "法于阴阳"的"法"意为"仿效、效法"，即遵循自然界的阴阳变化规律。《新牛津英汉双解大词典》对 abide 的解释为 accept or act in accordance with (a rule, decision, or recommendation)，即接受或者遵循某些行为规范和法则，其含义比 follow 更强。"阴阳"实际上指的是阴阳规律，译为 the principle of yin and yang。

引例 Citations:

◎上古之人，其知道者，法于阴阳，和于术数。（《素问·上古天真论》）

（上古时代的人，其中懂得养生之道的智者，能效法天地阴阳的变化规律，施行各种合宜的调养精气的方法。）

The wise man in remote antiquity who knew ways of health preservation abode by the principle of yin and yang, regulated and nourished essential qi with *Shushu* (methods and techniques of health preservation). (*Plain Conversation*)

◎始论乎天真，次论乎调神，既以法于阴阳，而继之以调于四气。（《丹溪心法附余》卷一）

（先论述质朴无邪的天性，其次论述调养精神，既要效法阴阳变化的规律，然后要调养四时之气。）

Unpretentious and innocent nature is expounded first before the discussion on regulating and cultivating spirit. It is important to abide by the principle of yin and yang, and then regulate life activities in accordance with climatic and phenological changes in the four seasons. (*Attached Supplements to "Danxi's Mastery of Medicine"*) hé yú shùshù

和于术数

Regulating and Nourishing Essential Qi with Shushu

施行各种合宜的调养精气的方法。术数，是以天文、历法、乐律等科学知识为基础，以"天人合一""天人感应"为理论，以阴阳五行学说为骨架，以人为的数字推演为手段，以种种方法观察自然界可注意的现象，并以此推知人事，趋吉避凶，推测人和国家的气数命运的方法或技术、手段。这里主要指导引、按跷等养生的方法。

The term means using various appropriate methods to regulate and nourish essential qi. *Shushu* (术数, literally techniques and numbers) refers to the methods or techniques with which people predict human affairs, bring good fortune and outcast evil as well as speculate the fate and destiny of people and states based on scientific knowledge including astronomy, calendar, and musical temperament. It is conducted in accordance with the theories of "oneness of heaven and human" and "interaction between heaven and human" within the framework of yin-yang theory and the five-element theory. Based on a set of rules about numbers that are arbitrarily defined, various methods are used for the observation of noticeable phenomena in nature. *Shushu* herein refers to ways of health preservation such as *daoyin* and massage.

【曾经译法】 /

【现行译法】 adjusting ways to cultivating health

【标准译法】 regulating and nourishing essential qi with *shushu*

【翻译说明】 "和于术数"指施行各种合宜的调养精气的方法。"和"表示"调和，调养"，译为 regulate and nourish，英文译法中需要补充"和"的对象"精气"。"术数"是各种方法的统称，无现成译法，宜采用音译。

引例 Citations:

◎上古之人，其知道者，法于阴阳，和于术数。（《素问·上古天真论》）

（上古时代的人，其中懂得养生之道的智者，能取法天地阴阳的变化规律，施行各种合宜的调养精气的方法。）

The wise man in remote antiquity who knew ways of health preservation abode by the principle of yin and yang, regulated and nourished essential qi with *shushu* (methods and techniques of health preservation). (*Plain Conversation*)

◎和，调也。术数者，调养精气之法也。（《黄帝内经素问集注》卷一）

（和，即调节。术数，即调养精气的方法。）

He (和) means regulation, while *shushu* means ways of regulating and nourishing essential qi. (*Collective Annotations of Plain Conversation in Yellow Emperor's Internal Canon of Medicine*)

◎术数所含甚广，如呼吸、按跷，及《四气调神论》养生、养收、养藏之道，《生气通天论》"阴平阳秘"，《阴阳应象大论》"七损八益"，《灵枢·本神》"长生久视"，本篇下文饮食起居之类。（《黄帝内经素问注证发微》）

（术数所包括的范围甚广，如呼吸吐纳、按跷，以及《四气调神大论》所论养生、养长、养收、养藏的方法，《生气通天论》所言"阴平阳秘"，《阴阳应象大论》所言"七损八益"，《灵枢·本神》所言"长生久视"，本篇下文所论饮食起居之类。）

Shushu is an umbrella term, including breathing and physical exercises such as inhalation and exhalation, massage, methods for preserving birth, growth, harvest, and storage discussed in "Major Discussion on Regulation of Spirit According to the Changes of the Four Seasons." It also includes the concept that "yin is stable and yang is compact" in "Discussion on Interrelationship between Life and Nature," "seven impairments and eight benefits" in "Major

Discussion on the Theory of Yin and Yang and the Corresponding Relationships Among All the Things in Nature," "long life with unfailing eyes and ears" in "Basic State of Spirit" of *Spiritual Pivot*, and diets as well as lifestyles covered in the following part of this text. (*Annotations and Commentary of Plain Conversation in Yellow Emperor's Internal Canon of Medicine*) qīsǔn bāyì

七损八益

Seven Impairments and Eight Benefits

古代七种损伤身体和八种有益于身体的性方法。长沙马王堆汉墓出土竹简《天下至道谈》明确记述了"七损八益"的内容，其文曰："八益：一曰治气，二曰致沫，三曰智（知）时，四曰畜气，五曰和沫，六曰窃（积）气，七曰寺（待）赢（盈），八曰定顷（倾）。七孙（损）：一曰闭，二曰泄，三曰竭，四曰勿，五曰烦，六曰绝，七曰费。"八种有益于人体的行为是调整呼吸、聚集唾液、掌握时机、保养元气、混合唾液、累积精气、保持精气满盈、精神镇定自若，七种有损于人体的行为是精道闭塞、精华漏泄、精力枯竭、所用不能、精神烦乱、截断失谐、疾速耗费。

The term refers to the seven harmful and eight beneficial ways of sex life in ancient times. According to the inscriptions on the bamboo slips, *Tian Xia Zhi Dao Tan* (*Discourse on the Utmost Method Under Heaven*), excavated in the Han Tombs at Mawangdui in Changsha, "The eight benefits are as follows: the first is regulating breathing; the second is promoting saliva; the third is understanding the proper time; the fourth is storing original qi; the fifth is harmonizing yin fluids; the sixth is accumulating essential qi; the seventh is maintaining abundance of essential qi, and the eighth is maintaining calm and balance. The seven impairments include internal blockage (suffering pain in sexual organs during the act), external leakage (perspiring during the act), exhaustion (consuming qi due to excessive engagement in the act), incompetence (impotence), vexation (feeling troubled and panting during the act), impasse (forcing oneself to engage in the act when the partner has no desire), and waste (performing the act in haste)." [1]

1　英文翻译参考：Douglas Wile. (1992). *Art of the Bedchamber: The Chinese Sexual Yoga Classics Including Women's Solo Meditation Texts*. New York: State University of New York Press. p81.

【曾经译法】INSUFFICIENCY OF SEVEN AND TONIFICATION OF EIGHT; seven harmful methods and eight favorable techniques in sexual life

【现行译法】sevenfold impairment and eightfold benefit; seven ills and eight benefits; seven impairments and eight benefits

【标准译法】seven impairments and eight benefits

【翻译说明】"七损八益"指的是七种损伤身体和八种有益于身体的性方法，因此采用直译的方法，即 seven impairments（七损）和 eight benefits（八益）。根据《新牛津英汉双解大词典》的释义，impairment 主要指对眼、耳、脑或肢体等的损伤。

引例 Citations:

◎能知七损八益，则二者可调；不知用此，则早衰之节也。（《素问·阴阳应象大论》）

（能够知道七损八益的方法，就可以调和阴阳；不懂得这个方法，人体就会过早地衰老。）

Yin and yang can be harmonized if the precepts of seven impairments and eight benefits are followed. Otherwise, people will age prematurely. (*Plain Conversation*)

◎能知七损八益，则阴不偏胜，阳不偏衰，故二者可调。（《素问悬解》卷一）

（能够知道七损八益的方法，就会使阴不偏盛而阳不偏衰，所以阴阳可以调和。）

Understanding seven impairments and eight benefits will help prevent yin from predominance and yang from deficiency, and hence the harmony between yin and yang can be achieved. (*Explanation of Unresolved Issues in "Plain Conversation"*)

◎人能慎保天真，待其二十方娶，守圣训七损八益之戒。(《医学一贯》)

（人能够谨慎地保养先天真气，等到了二十岁才结婚，坚守圣人告谕的七损八益的戒律。）

One can prudently maintain his congenital qi if he does not marry before age twenty and sticks to the precepts of seven impairments and eight benefits advanced by the sages. (*Consistent Medical Principles*) yīnshì lìdǎo

因势利导

Treatment in Accordance with the Tendency of Pathological Changes

顺着事情发展的趋势，向有利于实现目的的方向加以引导。中医学强调在治疗疾病的过程中，要综合考虑各种因素，顺应病程、病位、病势特点，以及阴阳消长、脏腑气血运行的规律，把握最佳时机，充分调动和利用机体"阴阳自和"的抗病、祛病、愈病的机制和能力，采取最适宜的方式加以治疗，推动其自主地进行自我调节，使阴阳、气血由失衡态转化为正常态。如根据病邪在上、在下、在表、在里等不同情况，分别选用涌吐、攻下、解表等方法治疗，从最简捷的途径，以最快的速度排出病邪，使正气不受或少受损伤，以最小的代价获得最佳的治疗效果。

The term refers to making things develop in a direction favorable to the accomplishment of goals in accordance with their trends in development. In traditional Chinese medicine, it is important to consider all factors in the treatment of diseases including the course, site, and characteristics of diseases and to comply with the theory of waxing and waning of yin and yang as well as the principle of qi and blood circulation in the zang-fu organs. It is also important to grasp the best time, to fully mobilize and exploit the physiological mechanism and human body's capacity of "spontaneous harmonization of yin and yang" in fighting, dispelling, and curing diseases, to adopt the most appropriate therapy for treatment, and to promote automatic self-regulation so that the balance of yin and yang, qi and blood can be restored. For example, according to different conditions of the diseases located in the upper, lower, exterior, or interior part of the human body, different therapies such as emesis, purgation, and relieving superficies can be used respectively to eliminate a disease in a simplest and fastest way. In doing so, no or less healthy qi is impaired and best outcomes can be achieved at the lowest cost.

【曾经译法】 treatment in accordance with the tendency of pathological changes

【现行译法】 treatment in accordance with tendency of pathological changes

【标准译法】 treatment in accordance with the tendency of pathological changes

【翻译说明】 "因势利导"强调在治疗疾病的过程中，根据疾病的各种变化因素，采用最合适的方法进行治疗。因此，该术语的翻译比较统一，均采用直译的方法，译为 treatment in accordance with the tendency of pathological changes。

引例 Citations:

◎痢疾之症……欲补其气，则邪气转加，欲清其火，则下行更甚。此时惟有因势利导之法，可行于困顿之间。(《石室秘录》卷二)

（痢疾病……想要补气的话，则邪气会增强；想要清火的话，则泻下会更剧烈。这时候只有采用因势利导的方法，才能解决这种艰难窘迫的境遇。）

In terms of treating diarrhea … Pathogenic qi will be enhanced if qi-supplementing method is used, and fire clearing may worsen symptoms of diarrhea. Only with the treatment in accordance with the tendency of pathological changes can such an intractable condition be relieved. (*Secret Records in Stone Room*)

◎脉沉者气多居里，故驱之使从下出为易，亦因势利导之法也。(《金匮要略心典》卷上)

（脉沉的患者，邪气多位于体内，因此采用泻下法祛除病邪较为容易，也是因势利导的方法。）

Patients with deep pulse have pathogenic qi inside their bodies. It would be relatively easier to treat them with purgative method to dispel pathogens, which fits with the treatment in accordance with the tendency of pathological changes.

◎疟发日早，为邪气上越于阳分，宜因势利导之，小柴胡加枳、桔。(《张氏医通》卷三)

（疟疾早上发作，是因为邪气向上位于阳分，应当采用因势利导之法，用小柴胡加枳壳、桔梗。）

The outbreak of malaria in the morning is due to the upper location of pathogens, which is in the yang phase. It should be treated in accordance with the tendency of pathological changes, administering *Xiao Chaihu* Decoction (Minor Bupleurum Decoction) with the addition of *zhiqiao* (*Fructus Aurantii*, orange fruit) and *jiegeng* (*Radix Platycodonis*, platycodon root). (*Comprehensive Medicine by Doctor Zhang Lu*) yǐ píng wéi qī

以平为期

Achieving Yin-yang Balance

以恢复人体阴阳相对平衡为治疗目标。中医学认为，人的各脏腑、组织之间，以及人与外界环境之间，若能维持相对的动态平衡，即可使各种生理活动正常地进行，而处于健康的状态；反之，人就会发生疾病。所以，从整体而言，所谓治病，就是纠偏求衡，协调人体内在环境及其与外界环境之间的关系，以求得新的平衡。除调整阴阳的偏盛、偏衰，恢复阴阳的相对平衡外，还包括针对气血不和、脏腑失调、升降失序等病理变化的调理，使之恢复和谐状态。

The term means the goal of the treatment is to restore the relative balance between yin and yang in human. In traditional Chinese medicine, physiological activities should work well to retain a healthy state if dynamic balance could be maintained among the zang-fu organs and tissues as well as between the person and the environment. Otherwise, diseases would occur. Therefore, holistically speaking, treating a disease is to rectify deviations and to coordinate the relationship between internal and external environment in order to keep a balance. Apart from adjusting the preponderance or deficiency of yin or yang to bring them back to normal, disharmony between qi and blood, zang-fu organs as well as disturbance in ascending and descending should be regulated to restore balance.

【曾经译法】

【现行译法】/

【标准译法】achieving yin-yang balance

【翻译说明】该术语在以往字典中均未被收录。"平"是指阴阳相对平衡，因此采用增译手段，翻译为 yin-yang balance。"期"意指目标。"以平为期"意思是以阴阳平衡为治疗目标；achieve 可

以表示通过努力、技能或勇气等获得，因此本术语翻译为
achieving yin-yang balance。

引例 Citations:

◎谨察阴阳所在而调之，以平为期。(《素问·至真要大论》)
　　(谨慎考察阴阳所处的部位然后进行调节，以恢复人体阴阳相对
　　平衡为治疗目标。)

To achieve yin-yang balance, careful observation on their location should be
made of yin and yang before regulation. (*Plain Conversation*)

◎治清以温，热而行之，以平为期，不可以过，此为大法。(《活人书》
卷六)
　　(治凉病用温药，药物趁热服用，以恢复人体阴阳相对平衡为目
　　的，不可以过度使用，这是治疗的关键。)

The medicine warm in property should be used in treating those diseases cold in
nature and taken when it is hot. The purpose is to achieve yin-yang balance and
not to overuse the medicine, which is the key to the treatment. (*Book for Saving
Lives*)

◎其为治者，泻实补虚，以平为期而已矣。(《儒门事亲》卷十三)
　　(这种治疗的核心是泻实补虚，以恢复人体阴阳相对平衡为
　　目的。)

The focus of the treatment is purging excess and supplementing deficiency,
with the purpose of achieving yin-yang balance in humans. (*Confucian's Duties
to Their Parents*)

司外揣内

Judging Internal Condition by Observing External Manifestations

通过观察事物的外在表象，来分析判断事物内在状况的认知方法，也称为以表知里。《孟子·告子下》说："有诸内必形诸外。"已认识到事物的本质和现象之间有着必然的联系，事物内在的变化，可通过某种方式在外部表现出来。故通过观察表象，可在一定程度上认识内在的变化机理。中医学通过对生命现象的观察、辨认，形成感性认识，进而发现并归纳本质属性的生命状态与表现于外在现象的固定联系，形成概念，完成对"象"的研究，即司外揣内之"司外"的阶段。然后由概念展开判断、推理，进入"揣内"阶段。揣，本质上是由现象形成概念，进而展开为判断、推理的逻辑思维过程。所以，"司外揣内"是为实现认识人体的"现象—状态"层面生命规律而采取的手段和思维途径。

The term, also known as "knowing the inside through the outside," refers to the cognitive method via which people judge internal condition by observing external manifestations. According to the section "Gaozi Part II" of *Mencius*, "the inside must be mirrored in the outside," denoting that people in ancient times had realized the interrelationship between essence and phenomenon and the internal changes could be manifested in external aspects. Therefore, by observing external manifestations, internal mechanism of changes can be understood up to a certain point. Through the observation on and identification of life phenomena, traditional Chinese medicine witnesses the development of perceptual cognition. It discovers and summarizes the fixed relationship between the nature of a living thing and its external condition. The concept is then established and the study of "manifestation" is completed, which is part of the work involved in "judging internal condition by observing external manifestations." The concept is further developed by identification and reasoning, reaching the level of "judging internal condition." "Judging" is essentially the logical thinking process from manifestation observation to concept development, involving making judgement and reasoning. Therefore, "judging internal condition by observing external manifestations" denotes the means and way of thinking adopted to understand the law of life at the "manifestation-condition" level in human.

【曾经译法】 /

【现行译法】 judging the inside by observation of the outside; predict the interior by inspecting the exterior; judging the inside from observation of the outside, inspecting exterior to predict interior

【标准译法】 judging internal condition by observing external manifestations

【翻译说明】 "外" 和 "内" 的译法一般为 the exterior/outside 和 the interior/inside。exterior 一般指建筑物等物体的外部；outside 泛指外部。这里的 "内、外" 指的是疾病的表象和本质，因此翻译为 internal condition 和 external manifestations 较好。"司" 的译法有 predict, judge 和 inspect。这里 "司" 更侧重于判断之后得出结论，因此 judge 较合适。

引例 Citations:

◎故远者司外揣内，近者司内揣外。(《灵枢·外揣》)

（所以从外部而言，观察病人的外在表现，可以推知内部的病变；从内部而言，通过所知病人的机体病变，可以推知外在的临床表现。）

From the external perspective, internal pathological changes can be judged by examining external manifestations of the patient. In turn, the external manifestations can be deduced by understanding the internal disorders of the zang-fu organs. (*Spiritual Pivot*)

◎视其外应，以知其内脏，则知所病矣。(《灵枢·本脏》)

    (观察他表现于外的情况，可以测知他的内脏变化，从而知道他所患的疾病。)

Observing external manifestations can provide health information of one's zang-fu organs and help predict the diseases that may occur. (*Spiritual Pivot*)

◎以我知彼，以表知里，以观过与不及之理。(《素问·阴阳应象大论》)

    (用自己的正常状态来比较病人的异常状态，从在表的症状去了解在里的病变，观察疾病偏盛与不足的病理。)

By comparing normal conditions of themselves with abnormal conditions of patients and by examining external manifestations, doctors gain an understanding of internal pathological changes. These are the methods they use to identify predominance and/or insufficiency of certain aspects. (*Plain Conversation*)

见微知著

Deducing Significant Changes from Subtle Signs

看到细微的苗头，就能推知可能发生的显著变化及结局，比喻小中见大。从中医对于疾病认识的角度而言，微，指微小、局部的变化；著，指明显的、整体的情况。见微知著，是指机体的某些局部的、微小的变化，常包含着整体的生理、病理信息，局部的细微变化常可反映出整体的状况，整体的病变可以从多方面表现出来。通过这些微小的变化，可以测知整体的情况。中医对脉、面、舌、耳等的诊察，都是这一原理的体现。

Subtle signs could indicate significant changes and outcomes that may occur. It figuratively means predicting the big from the small. According to traditional Chinese medicine, *wei* (微, subtle or tiny) refers to small, local changes in body parts and *zhu* (著, significant) refers to obvious, overall state of the body. The term means that local and minor changes can indicate the physiological and pathological information of the whole body, i.e., the overall condition is mirrored in local subtle changes as the diseases in whole body can be manifested in many aspects. By examining these subtle changes, the overall condition can be determined. Examinations of pulse, face, tongue, and ears are the applications of this principle in practice.

【曾经译法】 /

【现行译法】 /

【标准译法】 deducing significant changes from subtle signs

【翻译说明】 "微"指微小、局部的变化，译为 subtle signs；"著"指明显的、整体的情况，译为 significant changes；"知"表示根据事实推断，翻译为 deduce。

引例 Citations:

◎病至思治，末也。见微知著，弥患于未萌，是为上工。(《医学心悟》卷一)

    (病来了才想起治疗为下工。见微知著，消灭隐患于未萌芽状态，这就是高明的医生。)

Treating a disease when it occurs is what the inferior doctor does. The superior doctor could deduce significant changes from subtle signs and would nip potential risks in the bud. (*Medical Understanding*)

◎倘能见微知著，宁至相寻于覆辙耶。(《寓意草》卷二)

    (倘若能见微知著，难道会接连不断的犯前人失败的教训吗？)

If you can deduce significant changes when noticing subtle signs of a disease, will you repeat the mistakes of your predecessors? (*Yu Chang's Case Records and Treatments*)

◎古人治未病不治已病，知者见微知著，自当加意调摄为佳。(《静香楼医案》)

    (古人在还没有生病的时候就进行预防，而不是在生病之后才去治疗，懂得这个道理的人，见微知著，自然应该注重调养为上。)

The ancients put prevention first instead of treating patients when they fall ill. Those who understand this principle could predict significant changes of the diseases when noticing subtle signs; therefore, regulating and cultivating health is the best strategy. (*Case Records of Jingxiang Mansion*) yǐ cháng héng biàn

以常衡变

Discerning Changes by Measuring Against the Normal

在认识正常的基础上，辨别、发现太过、不及的异常变化。常，指健康的、生理的状态；变，指异常的、病理的状态。中医诊断疾病，强调首先应掌握正常人的健康状态，以正常人为标准，通过比较找出差别，进而认识疾病。如《素问·平人气象论》提出以健康人的呼吸与脉动关系为标准，以判断疾病之虚实，健康人的呼吸与脉动比率为一息脉动四次，若超过此比率为数脉，达不到此比率为迟脉。中医对人的面色、舌象的判断，均是采用以常衡变的方法。

Based on an understanding of the normal state, one can differentiate and discover abnormal changes such as excess or inadequacy. *Chang* (常, normal) refers to the healthy physiological state; *bian* (变, change) refers to the abnormal pathological state. According to traditional Chinese medicine (TCM) diagnosis, emphasis should be first laid upon knowing the healthy state of average people and taking the "normal" as the standard to identify differences and the disease. According to the section "Discussion on Qi Manifestation in a Healthy Person" of *Plain Conversation*, for example, excess and/or deficiency of a disease could be determined based on the relationship between the respiration and pulsing of a healthy person. For a healthy individual, the pulse beats four times in a cycle of exhalation and inhalation. If the ratio exceeds it, it is rapid pulse; if it is fewer than four times, it is slow pulse. Guided by the principle of discerning changes by measuring against the normal, TCM practitioners examine the complexion and the tongue of patients.

【曾经译法】/

【现行译法】/

【标准译法】discerning changes by measuring against the normal

【翻译说明】"常"指的是健康的、正常的生理状态，可以翻译为 the

normal;"变"是指异常的,病理的状态,可以翻译为 changes (act or process through which something becomes different)。"衡"可以翻译为 discern,表示辨别、识别 (recognize or find out)。"以常衡变"可译为 discerning changes by measuring against the normal。

引例 Citations:

◎平人者,不病也。常以不病调病人,医不病,故为病人平息以调之为法。(《素问·平人气象论》)

（所谓的平人,就是没有病的人。诊脉的法则是用无病的人的呼吸来诊测病人的脉率,医生是无病的人,所以调匀呼吸来诊测病人的脉搏次数。）

Healthy individuals are those who are not ill. The respiratory rate of a healthy individual is usually used as the criterion to measure the pulse conditions of sick people. Doctors are healthy individuals, so they can regulate their rate of breathing to examine the pulse beats of their patients. (*Plain Conversations*)

◎持脉之道,须明常变……先识常脉,而后可以察变脉。(《景岳全书·脉神章》)

（诊脉的规则,必须明晰以常衡变……先认识正常的脉象,然后才可以辨别异常的脉象。）

The principle of pulse-taking is to discern changes by measuring against the normal pulse... Normal pulse conditions should be well understood so that abnormalities can be identified. (*Jingyue's Complete Works*)

◎盖应者常也,不应者变也,知其常变,则知其病症矣。(《望诊遵经》)

（气色、脉象、症状相应者为常态，不应者为变异，懂得疾病的常与变，就可以知道所患的病症。）

When complexion, pulse condition, and other manifestations are in consistency, it is considered normal; if not, it is considered abnormal. By understanding the normal and abnormal states of the body, the doctor could diagnose the diseases. (*Principles Followed in Inspection Diagnosis*) yīn fā zhī shòu

因发知受

Disease Manifestations Help Determine the Cause.

根据机体在疾病中所反应的证候特征，确定疾病病因的风、寒、暑、湿、燥、火属性，而不是根据气候变化或气温、湿度高低做出判断。"发"指人在疾病中出现的证候表现，"受"指感受的邪气和机体的反应状态。各种外来的邪气作用于人体后，是否发病取决于邪正斗争的结果。邪气的性质主要是通过对证候的辨别确定的，如天气突然变化，并非所有的人都会感受外邪，是否感受外邪、感受何种邪气，主要是由机体的反应能力、反应状态决定的，必须通过人体表现的证候做出判断。这种探求病因的方法，也称为"审症求因"。也就是通过审察临床病变的各种表现推求疾病发生发展的内在机制和本质。

Doctors should determine the pathogenic factors, i.e., wind, cold, summer-heat, dampness, dryness, and fire, based on the manifested disease pattern rather than climate change, temperature, or humidity. *Fa* (发, manifestation) refers to the signs and symptoms of the pattern that occur. *Shou* (受, receiving) refers to the pathogenic qi that one is affected and the responses that one's body makes. Whether the disease occurs or not after various pathogenic qi affects the body depends on the result of the fight between healthy qi and pathogenic qi. The nature of pathogenic qi is mainly determined through the differentiation of a pattern. For example, when the weather suddenly changes, not everyone will be affected by external pathogens. Whether and by what kind of pathogenic qi one is affected are mainly determined by one's body's ability and condition to cope with pathogens, and these must be diagnosed according to the signs and symptoms manifested in the body. This method of identifying the cause is also described as "examining symptoms to identify the cause," i.e., to understand the internal mechanism and the nature of disease development by examining the signs and symptoms.

【曾经译法】 assess the patterns and seek the cause; seek the cause from patterns identified (注：对应"审症求因")

【现行译法】 seeking the cause from symptoms; determining the cause of the disease according to the clinical manifestations; differentiating syndrome to identify cause; identification of cause according to syndrome differentiation (注：以上皆对应"审症求因")

【标准译法】 Disease manifestations help determine the cause.

【翻译说明】 "因发知受"指根据症状特点来判断病因，manifestation 侧重表示疾病的外在表现，短语 clinical manifestations 常用来表示临床特征。按照术语结构语序，"因发知受"意译为 Disease manifestations help determine the cause。

引例 Citations:

◎外邪之感，受本难知，发则可辨，因发知受。(《伤寒溯源集》卷一)
（到底感受了哪种外邪，是很难推测的，发病后就可以辨别了，根据机体在疾病中所反应的证候特征，就可以确定疾病的病因。）

It is hard to surmise what kind of external pathogen affects the human body before the onset of a disease is shown. It can be identified after the disease occurs. Manifestations could help determine the cause of the disease. (*Tracing Cold Damage to Its Source*)

◎观其脉证，知犯何逆，随证治之。(《伤寒论》)
（通过诊察患者的脉象和症状，可以推测感受了哪种病邪，根据其证候而治疗。）

An examination of the pulse and other symptoms can help identify the cause of the disease and the treatment should be given in accordance with the pattern. (*Treatise on Cold Damage*) sìzhěn hécān

四诊合参

Synthesis of Four Diagnostic Methods

望、闻、问、切四诊并重，相参互证，综合考虑所收集的病情资料，以得出更为准确的诊断。疾病是一个复杂的过程，其临床表现可体现于多个方面且千变万化，而望、闻、问、切四诊是从不同的角度了解病情和收集临床资料，各有其独特的方法与意义，不能互相取代，若仅以单一的诊法进行诊察，势必造成资料收集的片面性，对诊断的准确性产生影响。因此，若要保证临床资料的全面、准确、详尽，必须强调各种诊法的合参互证与补充。

The four equally important diagnostic methods are used for cross reference, including inspection, listening and smelling, inquiry, as well as pulse-taking and palpation. The collected information of the diseases should be considered thoroughly in order to make an accurate diagnosis. Disease is a complex process and its clinical manifestations can be reflected in various aspects and may change from time to time. The four diagnostic methods are adopted to understand the diseases and help collect the relevant information from different perspectives, each with its unique technique and value. They cannot replace each other. If only one single method is used, it will inevitably lead to the one-sidedness of data collection, which will affect the accuracy of diagnosis. Therefore, in order to obtain comprehensive, accurate, and detailed clinical data, it is more than necessary to emphasize the combined use of four diagnostic methods and they should supplement one another.

【曾经译法】 comprehensive analysis by the four examination methods; DEDUCTION BY THE FOUR DIAGNOSTIC TECHNIQUES; comprehensive analysis by four methods of examination; comprehensive diagnosis by four methods; correlate all four examination; correlation of all four examinations

【现行译法】comprehensive analysis of the data obtained by the four diagnostic techniques; comprehensive consideration of the four examinations; synthesis of four diagnostic method; comprehensive diagnosis by four methods; comprehensive analysis of the data obtained from the four examinations; synthesis of the four diagnostics; correlation of all four examinations; comprehensive analysis of four examinations

【标准译法】synthesis of four diagnostic methods

【翻译说明】四诊指望、闻、问、切四种诊断方法，译为 four diagnostic methods。synthesis 强调不同方法的有机综合运用，comprehensive 突出"包含各个方面的综合体"。"四诊合参"强调四种诊法的运用需要有机结合，因此 synthesis 比 comprehensive analysis 更合适。

引例 Citations:

◎观清浊以辨阴阳，视微甚以知虚实，四诊合参，其庶几乎？（《望诊遵经》）

（观察面色的清浊可以辨别疾病的阴阳属性，通过诊察病人面部颜色的深浅以了解疾病的虚实，四诊相参互证，应该就差不多了吧？）

Examination of facial complexion in terms of freshness or turbidity could help identify yin or yang property of the disease; examination in terms of dark or light color could help determine deficiency or excess nature of the disease. The synthesis of four diagnostic methods cannot go wrong, can it? (*Principles Followed in Inspection Diagnosis*)

◎上士欲会其全，非备四诊不可。（《濒湖脉学》）

（高明的医生想要全面把握病情，必须四诊并重，相参互证。）

Superior doctors should value all four diagnostic methods when they aspire to understand the disease comprehensively. (*Binhu Study on Pulses*)

三部九候

Three Sections and Nine Manifestations

三部九候诊法，是指对头、手、下肢三部之动脉进行切按，以诊察疾病的诊脉方法。此法首见于《素问·三部九候论》，切脉的部位有头（上）、手（中）、下肢（下）三部，每部又分为天、人、地三部，合为九候。上部天，是指两侧颞动脉，可以反映头额及颞部的病痛；上部人，是指耳前动脉，可以了解目和耳的情况；上部地，是指两颊动脉，可以了解口腔与牙齿的情况。中部天，是手太阴肺经的动脉处，可候肺气；中部人，是手少阴心经的动脉处，可候心气；中部地，是手阳明大肠经的动脉处，可候胸中之气。下部天，是足厥阴肝经的动脉处，候肝气；下部人，是足太阴脾经或足阳明胃经的动脉处，候脾胃之气；下部地，是足少阴肾经的动脉处，候肾气。后世以寸口脉（参见下一词条）的寸、关、尺为三部，三部各有浮、中、沉为九候，也称为三部九候。

The term refers to the pulse-taking method of feeling the arterial pulse of the head, hands and feet to diagnose diseases. It was first described in the section "Discussion on Three Sections and Nine Manifestations" of *Plain Conversation*. The arteries of the three sections, i.e., head (upper), hand (middle), and foot (lower), are palpated and each section is further divided into three subsections, namely, heaven, human, and earth, making nine sections altogether. The upper-section heaven refers to the temporal arteries on both sides, which can indicate the pain in the forehead and temples; the upper-section human, the anterior auricular artery, can reveal the condition of the eyes and the ears; the upper-section earth, the cheek arteries, can manifest the condition of the mouth and teeth. The middle-section heaven refers to the artery of the Lung Meridian of Hand-*taiyin*, where the condition of lung qi can be manifested; the middle-section human refers to the artery of the Heart Meridian of Hand-*shaoyin*, where the condition of heart qi can be detected; the middle-section earth refers to the artery of the Large Intestine Meridian of Hand-*yangming*, where the condition of chest qi can be revealed. The lower-section heaven is the artery of the Liver Meridian of Foot-*jueyin*, which can reflect the condition of liver qi; the lower-section human refers to the artery of the Spleen Meridian of Foot-*taiyin* or the Stomach Meridian of Foot-*yangming*, which can indicate the condition of spleen qi and stomach qi; the lower-section earth is the artery of the Kidney Meridian of Foot-*shaoyin*, which can reveal the condition of kidney qi. Later generations adopt *cunkou* diagnostic method (see the following entry), taking *cun* (寸), *guan* (关), and *chi* (尺) as the three sections for pulse-taking. Then pulse-taking at each section is divided into three different aspects according to the force, i.e., light, medium, and heavy, thus making a total of nine manifestations. This is also described as three sections and nine manifestations.

【曾经译法】 three regions and their nine subdivisions for pulse-feeling; three regions and nine modes; three regions and nine locations for pulse feeling; three portions and nine pulse-takings; three positions and nine indicators

【现行译法】 three portions and nine pulse-taking; nine readings of three sections; three regions, three portions (for pulse taking); three portions and nine positions for pulse-taking; nine readings on three sections; three positions and nine indicators; three positions and nine pulse-takings

【标准译法】 three sections and nine manifestations

【翻译说明】 "三部"指头、手和足，每部又分天、地和人，共为"九候"。"三部"的译法有 three regions, three portions 和 three sections。portion 释义是 one part of something larger，常指总体中的一部分 ; region 的意思是 a large area of land, usually without exact limit。因此 section 更合适，表示界限分明、相对独立的部分（any of the parts into which something is divided）。"候"的译法有 locations, modes, pulse-takings, readings 和 positions。根据中文释义，应该指的是"征候，征象"，因此翻译为 manifestations。

引例 Citations:

◎故人有三部，部有三候，以决死生，以处百病，以调虚实，而除邪疾。
（《素问·三部九候论》）

　　（所以人的脉有三部，每部各有三候，根据它去决定死生，诊断
　　百病，调治虚实，祛除病邪。）

Therefore, there are three sections for pulse-taking in the human body and each
section is divided into three subsections, which are examined to determine
prognosis, diagnose diseases, and relieve deficiency and/or excess to remove
diseases. (*Plain Conversation*)

◎参伍不调者病，三部九候皆相失者死。（《素问·三部九候论》）

　　（脉搏错乱不相协调的主患病，三部九候都失其常度的主死症。）

Irregular and disharmonic pulse signifies impending diseases. If all the nine
manifestations on three sections are in disharmony, it indicates impending
death. (*Plain Conversation*)

◎脉有三部九候，各何所主之？然：三部者，寸关尺也；九候者，浮中沉
也。（《难经·十八难》）

　　（寸口脉诊有三部九候的诊法，各部分别所主候哪些部位的疾病
　　呢？回答说：三部是指寸、关、尺，九候是指每一部脉又有浮取、
　　中取、沉取的方法。）

The *cunkou* diagnostic method means the examination of three sections and
nine manifestations. What does each mean? Here is the answer: the three
sections refer to *cun*, *guan*, and *chi*; the nine manifestations refer to the
results obtained by taking pulse using three different levels of force, i.e., light,
medium, and heavy, respectively. (*Canon of Difficult Issues*)

cùnkǒu zhěnfǎ

寸口诊法

Cunkou Diagnostic Method

切按桡骨茎突内侧一段桡动脉的搏动，根据其脉动形象，以推测人体生理、病理状态的一种诊察方法。通常以桡骨茎突为标记，其内侧的部位为关，关前（腕侧）为寸，关后（肘侧）为尺。两手各有寸、关、尺三部，共六部脉，寸、关、尺三部又可施行浮、中、沉三候。寸口三部所分候脏腑，其中左寸候心，右寸候肺，并统括胸以上及头部的疾病；左关候肝胆，右关候脾胃，并统括膈以下至脐以上部位的疾病；两尺候肾，并包括脐以下至足部的疾病。此外，也有不分寸、关、尺，但以浮、中、沉分候脏腑的方法，如以左手浮取候心，中取候肝，沉取候肾；右手浮取候肺，中取候脾，沉取候肾（命门）。

The term refers to the diagnostic method of feeling the pulse at the radial artery in the medial side of the styloid, through which the doctor could determine the physiological and pathological states of a human body. A prominent bone, i.e., styloid process of the radius, marks the section. The medial part of it is *guan* (关); in the front of *guan* (to the wrist) is *cun* (寸), and at the back of *guan* (to the elbow) is *chi* (尺). There are three sections on each hand and therefore six in total. At the sections of *cun*, *guan*, and *chi*, pulse can be taken respectively with three different levels of force, i.e., light, medium, and heavy. Each section is believed to correspond to one of the zang-fu organs. C*un* on the left hand corresponds to the heart; *cun* on the right hand, the lung, including the parts above the chest and the head as well. *Guan* on the left hand corresponds to the liver and the gallbladder; *guan* on the right hand, the spleen and stomach, including the parts between the diaphragm and the umbilicus. *Chi* on both hands corresponds to the kidney, including the parts in between the umbilicus and the feet. Instead of using *cun*, *guan*, and *chi*, one can examine the conditions of the zang-fu organs according to the applied force in three levels, i.e., light, medium, and heavy. For example, on the left hand, light force, medium force, and heavy force are used to identify the condition of the heart, the liver, and the kidney, respectively. On the right hand, they are used to identify the condition of the lung, the spleen, and the kidney (life gate), respectively.

【曾经译法】 /

【现行译法】 wrist pulse-taking method; *cun* pulse-taking method

【标准译法】 *cunkou* diagnostic method

【翻译说明】 2000 年以前，大部分字典都将"寸口"直接音译，写作 *cun kou* 或者 *cunkou*。2000 年以后出版的字典逐渐开始用 wrist (a joint connecting the hand with the forearm)。考虑到术语的文化特色和回译性，"寸口诊法"翻译为 *cunkou* diagnostic method 较妥。

引例 Citations:

◎此论在诊脉察色调尺之中，则是寸口诊法也。(《扁鹊脉书难经》卷一)

　　(这一论述在诊脉、观察面色和诊察尺肤之中，就是寸口诊法。)

In the discourse on pulse-taking, examination of facial complexion, and inspecting the skin from the elbow to the wrist, the statement refers to *cunkou* diagnostic method. (*Bianque's Canon of Difficult Issues on Pulse-taking*)

◎今则止用寸口诊法，不为不妙。(《类经》卷六)

　　(现在只用寸口脉诊法，是非常巧妙的。)

It is ingenious to only adopt *cunkou* diagnostic method at present. (*Classified Classic*) biànzhèng lùnzhì

辨证论治

Pattern Differentiation and Treatment

运用中医学理论辨析有关疾病的资料以确定证名，并制定出相应治疗措施的思维和实践过程，可分为辨证和论治两个阶段。所谓辨证，就是将望、闻、问、切等诊法所收集的资料、症状和体征，在中医理论指导下，通过分析综合，辨清疾病的原因、性质、部位及邪正之间的关系等，最后概括、判断为某种性质的证。辨证的过程，就是从机体反应性的角度来认识疾病，分析疾病当时所表现的症状和体征，以认识这些临床表现的内在联系，并且以此来反映疾病该阶段本质的临床思维过程。论治，则是根据辨证的结果，确定相应的治疗原则和方法，选择适当的治疗手段和措施来处理疾病的思维和实践过程。

The term refers to the thinking process and the practice of differentiating the patterns based on the collected data and formulating the corresponding treatment plan in accordance with the theory of traditional Chinese medicine (TCM). It involves two stages: pattern differentiation and treatment. The former means collecting data as well as signs and symptoms through the four diagnostic methods (inspection, listening and smelling, inquiry, as well as pulse-taking and palpation) and making a comprehensive analysis of information to differentiate the cause, nature, and location of the disease and then to identify the relationship between pathogenic qi and healthy qi under the guidance of TCM theory. One is expected to eventually generalize the data to a pattern of certain nature. Such is the logical thinking process of understanding the disease from the perspective of body's responses. Analyzing clinical manifestations helps one identify their internal relationships, based on which the nature of the disease can be determined at a certain stage. The latter involves determining the corresponding treatment principle and methods based on pattern differentiation and opting for appropriate therapies to remove diseases.

【曾经译法】 BIANZHEN LUNZHI (PLANNING TREATMENT ACCORDING TO DIAGNOSIS); selection of treatment based on the differential diagnosis; treatment based on syndrome differentiation; identify patterns and determine treatment; determine treatment by patterns identified; diagnosis and treatment based on the overall analysis of signs and symptoms; treatment with syndrome differentiation

【现行译法】 selection of treatment according to differential diagnosis; treatment based on syndrome differentiation; syndrome differentiation and treatment; pattern identification; syndrome differentiation and treatment; pattern identification and treatment

【标准译法】 pattern differentiation and treatment

【翻译说明】 "辨证"的意思是通过分析最后判断为某种证，曾经采用的译法有 syndrome differentiation, pattern identification 以及音译。译词 syndrome 对应西医的"综合征"，中医的"证"只是指患者表现出来的一系列相互关联的证候，目前通常用 pattern 表示。译词 differentiation 强调"辨别"，identification 强调"确认"，因此前者更合适。"辨证论治"可分为辨证和论治两个阶段，翻译成 pattern differentiation and treatment 较为合适。

引例 Citations:

◎不明六气变化之理、辨证论治，岂能善哉。(《医门棒喝》卷三)
（不了解风、寒、暑、湿、燥、火六气变化的道理以及辨证论治的方法，怎么能好呀？）

How could the disease be cured if the doctor did not know the theory of six qi (wind, cold, summer-heat, dampness, dryness, and fire) or the principle of treating diseases based on pattern differentiation? (*Medical Warnings*)

◎诚以汉唐家法，辨证论治，具有精义，可为万世不易之法守。(《中风斠诠》序)

　　　　(的确以汉唐时期师徒传授的学风，辨证论治，具有精深奥义，可以作为万世不变的法则。)

Pattern differentiation and treatment, as the tradition of study style inherited from the master to the apprentice in the Han and Tang dynasties, is indeed profound and can be the eternal principle to follow. (*Fair Interpretation of Wind Stroke*)

◎仲景立言……开后学辨证施治之法门。(《伤寒溯源集》卷一)

　　　　(张仲景著书立说……开启了后世学者辨证施治的门径。)

Zhang Zhongjing wrote books to expound his theories... (He) was the first physician to advance the idea of pattern differentiation and treatment for later scholars to abide by. (*Tracing Cold Damage to Its Source*) tóngbìng yìzhì

同病异治

Different Treatments for the Same Disease

同病异治是指同一疾病，不同发展阶段所表现的证候不同，或因其地域、气候、体质等因素的影响，所表现的证候有差异，而采取不同的方法治疗。如麻疹，由于病理发展的阶段不同，因而治疗方法也不一样。初起麻疹未透，宜发表透疹；中期多肺热显著，常须清肺；后期多为余热未尽，肺胃阴伤，则须以养阴清热为主。

The term means that the same disease should be treated with different approaches according to different patterns manifested at different stages or resulting from variations in such factors as geography, climate, and body constitution. Take measles for example. The treatment should vary according to the pathological development at different stages. In the early stage, the rash is not fully developed and the treatment should be resolving superficies to promote eruption. In the mid stage, lung heat is always prominent, so it is important to clear the lung. In the late stage, remaining heat is always present and impairs lung yin and stomach yin, which requires nourishing yin and clearing heat.

【曾经译法】 treating the same disease with different methods; different treatments for the same disease

【现行译法】 treating the same disease with different methods; different treatments for the same disease

【标准译法】 different treatments for the same disease

【翻译说明】 "同病异治"指同一疾病在不同的证候阶段采取不同的治疗方法，各词典中给出的译法比较趋同：treat the same disease with different methods。考虑到简洁性和术语突出的是"异治"部分，将"同病异治"译为 different treatments for the same disease。

引例 Citations:

◎夫痈气之息者，宜以针开除去之；夫气盛血聚者，宜石而泻之，此所谓同病异治也。(《素问·病能论》)

（由于气结停聚而成的痈肿，应该用针刺开其穴，泻去其气；若气盛血聚，脓已成熟的痈肿，应该用砭石泻其瘀血，这就是所说的同病异治。）

Neck carbuncle due to the stagnation of qi can be treated with acupuncture to disperse qi. Cases with formed pus due to predominance of qi and coagulation of blood can be treated with stone needle to remove static blood. Such treatments are known as different treatments for the same disease. (*Plain Conversation*)

◎西北之气散而寒之，东南之气收而温之，所谓同病异治也。(《素问·五常政大论》)

（西北方气候寒冷，应该散其外寒，清其里热；东南方气候温热，应该收敛外散的阳气，温散内寒，这就是所说的同病异治。）

It is cold in the northwest, so the treatment should concentrate on dissipating cold and clearing interior heat; it is warm in the southeast, so the treatment should focus on astringing the leakage of yang qi and dissipating interior cold by warming. This is described as different treatments for the same disease. (*Plain Conversation*) yìbìng tóngzhì

异病同治

Same Treatment for Different Diseases

异病同治是指不同的疾病，在其发展演变的过程中，有时可以出现相同或近似的病理变化，表现出相同或近似的证，故可采用相同的方法予以治疗。如慢性肠炎、肾炎、哮喘，病虽不同，但在它们的发展过程中，都可以出现肾阳虚的病理变化，故均可用温补肾阳的方法予以治疗。

The term means that different diseases could be treated with the same method when they manifest the same or similar pathological change or disease pattern in their development. For example, such diseases as chronic enteritis, nephritis, and asthma could be treated with the same method of warming and tonifying kidney yang since all of them show the pathological change of kidney-yang deficiency in their progression.

【曾经译法】 treat the different diseases with the same method; treating different diseases with same therapy; treating different diseases with the same method; like treatment of unlike disease; the same treatment for different diseases

【现行译法】 treating different diseases with the same therapeutic principle; same treatment for different diseases; treating different diseases with the same therapy; treating different diseases with the same method

【标准译法】 same treatment for different diseases

【翻译说明】 "异病同治"指不同的疾病呈现相同的病理变化时采取相同的治疗方法，各词典中给出的译法比较趋同：treat different diseases with the same method。考虑到简洁性和术语突出的是"同治"部分，将"异病同治"译为 same treatment for different diseases。

引例 Citations:

◎与热病之邪伏少阴，热伤胃汁，火迫心包不殊，故可异病同治。(《张氏
医通》卷二)

（与热病邪气潜伏少阴，热邪耗伤胃阴，火邪内侵心包相同，所
以可以异病同治。）

This disease is like the following conditions: pathogenic qi of the febrile disease remains dormant in the *shaoyin* meridian, pathogenic heat consumes stomach yin, and pathogenic fire invades the pericardium. Therefore, all of them could be treated with the same method. (*Comprehensive Medicine by Doctor Zhang Lu*)

◎治之者，或同病异治，或异病同治。(《神灸经纶》卷三)

（治疗这类病证，或者同病异治，或者异病同治。）

For these diseases, either the rule of different treatments for the same disease or the principle of same treatment for different diseases should be followed. (*Rules and Principles of Moxibustion*) hányīn hányòng

寒因寒用

Treating Cold with Cold

反治法之一。用寒凉性质的药物治疗表象为寒的病证的治法。此法适用于里热极盛，阻遏阳气不能外达，外有若干假寒征象的真热假寒证。如热厥证，阳热内盛，热邪深伏于里，常表现出壮热、恶热、烦渴饮冷、尿赤、脉数等里热征象；同时，由于里热盛极，阻遏阳气不能外达，而见手足逆冷、脉沉等假寒之象，治疗须用寒凉性质的药物清其内热以治本，则假寒的现象自可消除。

The term refers to one of the paradoxical treatments, meaning using cold-natured medicinals to treat the diseases with cold signs and symptoms. This method is applicable to relieving the pattern of true heat with pseudo-cold manifestations due to exuberant interior heat preventing yang qi from reaching out to the skin. Take heat syncope for example. On the one hand, internal yang heat is predominant and pathogenic heat is hidden deep inside, showing symptoms of interior heat such as high fever, aversion to heat, vexation, thirst with a desire for cold drinks, dark urine, and rapid pulse. On the other hand, the extremely predominant interior heat prevents yang qi from flowing outward and causes pseudo-cold manifestations such as reversal cold of the limbs and deep pulse. In this case, medicinals cold and/or cool in nature should be used to clear the internal heat to remove the root cause of the disease, thus having the pseudo-cold symptoms relieved accordingly.

【曾经译法】 treating the pseudo-cold diseases with drugs of cold nature; treating cold with cold; using medicines of cold nature to treat pseudo-cold syndrome

【现行译法】 using drugs of cold nature to treat pseudo-cold syndrome; using cold for cold; treating false cold syndrome with cold herbs; using herbs of cold nature to treat pseudo-cold syndrome; using cold when the cause is cold; treat cold with cold; treating cold with cold

【标准译法】 treating cold with cold

【翻译说明】 "寒因寒用"指用寒凉性质的药物治疗表象为寒的病症。"寒因"指的是表面有寒象，实为内热的疾病，译为 use drugs/medicine of cold nature to treat pseudo-cold pattern/syndrome 是符合术语内涵的。但考虑到简洁性和回译性，并且体现"寒因寒用"是中医治则之一，本书倾向于翻译为 treating cold with cold。

引例 Citations:

◎热因热用，寒因寒用……必伏其所主，而先其所因。(《素问·至真要大论》)

　　(用热性药物治疗表象为热的病证，用寒性药物治疗表象为寒的病证……要制伏其主病，必先找出致病的原因。)

Treat heat with heat, and treat cold with cold... To cure a disease, the cause must be made clear first. (*Plain Conversation*)

◎或寒因寒用，热因热用，因事制宜，用无不当。(《幼幼集成》)

　　(或者用寒性药物治疗表象为寒的病证，用热性药物治疗表象为热的病证，根据不同的事情，制定适宜的治法，使用就没有不合适之处。)

Or treat cold with cold; treat heat with heat. Either is appropriate if treatment is given in accordance with specific conditions. (*Compendium of Pediatrics*)

热因热用

Treating Heat with Heat

反治法之一。用温热性质的药物治疗其表象为热的病证的治法。如少阴病阴寒内盛，临床见下利清谷，手足厥逆，脉微欲绝；但由于阴盛格阳，而又见面色赤、身反不恶寒等假热现象，治疗用温热的通脉四逆汤顺从表热之象而违逆其阴寒之本。又如气虚发热之证，因脾胃阳气虚损，水谷精气当升不升，反下流于下焦，化为阴火，阴火上扰而发热，治疗用甘温之补中益气汤，升发脾阳，升举下陷精气，即甘温除热法，亦属热因热用之例。

The term refers to one of the paradoxical treatments, meaning using medicinal of hot nature to treat the diseases with heat manifestations. Take *shaoyin* disease with excessive internal yin-cold for example. Its clinical manifestations include diarrhea with undigested food, reversal cold of the extremities, as well as faint and impalpable pulse. However, pseudo-heat signs and symptoms such as "red complexion" and "no aversion to cold" can be present due to exuberant yin repelling yang. Therefore, *Tongmai Sini* Decoction (Decoction for Treating Cold Limbs by Promoting Vessels) of warm-hot nature is adopted in compliance with the exterior heat but in conflict with the root cause of yin cold. Another example is the qi-deficiency pattern with fever. Due to the deficiency of yang qi of the spleen and the stomach, the essence derived from food and drinks fails to ascend but descends instead to the lower energizer and transforms into yin fire which disturbs upwards and causes fever. *Buzhong Yiqi* Decoction (Decoction for Tonifying Middle Energizer and Boosting Qi) of sweet-warm property should be used to ascend spleen yang (qi) and raise the sinking essential qi, which is described as removing fever with medicinals sweet in flavor and warm in property. This is also an example of treating heat with heat.

【曾经译法】 treat the pseudo-heat syndrome with drugs of hot nature; treating heat with heat; treating pseudo-heat diseases with drugs of hot nature; using herbs of hot nature to treat pseudo-heat syndrome

【现行译法】 using warm-natured drugs to treat pseudo-heat syndrome; using heat for heat; treating pseudo-heat syndrome with hot therapy; using heat when the cause is heat; treat heat with heat

【标准译法】 treating heat with heat

【翻译说明】 "热因热用"指用温热性质的药物治疗表象为热的病症。"热因"指的是表面呈热象，实为内寒的疾病，译为 use drugs/medicine of hot nature to treat pseudo-heat pattern/syndrome 是符合术语内涵的。但考虑到简洁性和回译性，并且体现"热因热用"是中医治则之一，本书倾向于翻译为 treating heat with heat。

引例 Citations:

◎热因热用，寒因寒用……必伏其所主，而先其所因。(《素问·至真要大论》)

（用热性药物治疗表象为热的病证，用寒性药物治疗表象为寒的病证……要制伏其主病，必先找出致病的原因。）

Treat heat with heat, and treat cold with cold... To cure a disease, the cause must be made clear first. (*Plain Conversation*)

◎或疑补中益气何以治热，殊不知热因热用，温能除热之理。(《济阳纲目》卷二十五)

（或者怀疑补中益气汤为什么能治疗发热，竟不知道"热因热用"，温性药物能够治疗发热的道理。）

Some people question why *Buzhong Yiqi* Decoction (Decoction for Tonifying Middle Energizer and Boosting Qi) could treat fever. It is surprising that they know nothing about the principle of treating heat with heat, i.e., medicine of warm nature could relieve fever. (*Guide to Saving Yang*) tōngyīn tōngyòng

通因通用

Treating the Flowing by Promoting Flow

　　反治法之一。用通利药物治疗具有泄泻等通利症状的实性病证的治法。此法适用于实邪内阻所致的通泻之证。如燥热内结，泄利粪水的"热结旁流"证，急用承气汤类方攻下燥实。《伤寒论》说："少阴病，自利清水，色纯青，心下必痛，口干燥者，可下之，宜大承气汤。"宿食内停，阻滞肠胃，致腹痛、肠鸣、泄泻，泻下物臭如腐败的鸡蛋，治以消食导滞攻下，荡涤积滞；瘀血所致崩漏，夹有血块，腹痛拒按，或产后瘀血内阻，恶露不尽，治宜活血化瘀；湿热蕴结膀胱所致的尿频、尿急、尿痛等淋证，治以清热利湿通淋。另如湿热蕴结大肠的痢疾，虽日下十余次，治疗仍不宜止涩，当清热通肠，调气行血。

The term refers to one of the paradoxical treatments, meaning treating the excess pattern with "flowing" disorders such as diarrhea using medicinals of unblocking function. This method is applicable to relieving diarrhea due to the internal retention of excessive pathogenic factors. For example, the pattern of "heat fecaloma with watery discharge" characterized by internal dryness-heat retention and diarrhea should be treated with *Chengqi* Decoction (Decoction for Purging Digestive Qi) to relieve dryness excess. According to *Treatise on Cold Damage*, "*Shaoyin* disease, characterized by spontaneous watery diarrhea of a greenish color, manifests pain below the heart. If the mouth is parched, purgative method can be used. *Da Cheng qi* Decoction (Major Decoction for Purging Digestive Qi) is appropriate." Other examples are as follows. When there is food retention in the stomach and intestines causing stomachache, borborygmus, and diarrhea with a foul stench of rotten eggs, it requires promoting digestion and purging stagnation. When there is metrorrhagia or metrostaxis with blood clots due to blood stasis and abdominal pain which is aggravated by pressure, or postpartum blood stagnation and lochiorrhea, it needs promoting blood circulation to remove stagnation. In terms of dampness-heat accumulation in the urinary bladder causing frequent, urgent, and painful urination, the method of clearing heat, draining dampness, and relieving stranguria should be adopted. For the dysentery due to dampness-heat accumulation in the large intestine which results in serious diarrhea for more than ten times a day, the treatment should be clearing heat to remove intestinal obstruction and regulating qi to promote blood circulation instead of astringing.

【曾经译法】 treat the diarrhetic diseases with cathartics; treating diarrhea by purgation; treating diarrhea with cathartics; using purgative method to treat unconfinedness; treating the stopped by stopping; treating diarrhea with purgatives

【现行译法】 treating discharging disease with purgatives; opening for the opened; using dredging method when the cause is incontinence; treat diarrhea with purgative; treating the unstopped by unstopping; treating incontinent syndrome with dredging method; treat dredging with dredging

【标准译法】 treating the flowing by promoting flow

【翻译说明】 "通因通用"中的第一个"通"的译法有 diarrhea, unconfinedness, discharging diseases, the cause is incontinence 和 dredging, 其中, dredge 表示清除河床的泥、草等, discharge 意思是排出, discharging diseases 的用法不多见。第二个"通"指的是用通利药物, 译为 purgatives, purgation, dredging 或 the unstopping 等, 其中 purgation 强调清除。"通因通用"指用通利药物治疗有通利症状的实证, 包括治疗泄泻、痢疾、淋证、崩漏等涉及水液、尿液、血液流动等病症, 考虑到简洁性和回译性, 建议译为 treating the flowing by promoting flow。

引例 Citations:

◎帝曰: 反治何谓? 岐伯曰: 热因热用, 寒因寒用, 塞因塞用, 通因通用。

（《素问·至真要大论》）

> （黄帝问道：反治怎么讲呢？岐伯回答说：用热性药物治疗表象为热的病证，用寒性药物治疗表象为寒的病证，用补益药物治疗虚性闭塞不通的病证，用通利的药物治疗实性通泻的病证。）

The Yellow Emperor asked: "What does paradoxical treatment mean?" Qibo answered: "Paradoxical treatment means treating heat with heat, treating cold with cold, treating the blocked by blocking, and treating the flowing by promoting flow." (*Plain Conversation*)

◎里急后重，数至圊而不便，宜通因通用。（《儒门事亲》卷一）

> （腹部窘迫，时时欲泻，肛门重坠，便出不爽，频繁到厕所但难以排便者，宜用"通因通用"的治法。）

The method of "treating the flowing by promoting flow" should be used in the case of tenesmus with frequent visits to the toilet and difficulty in defecation. (*Confucians' Duties to Their Parents*)

◎下痢……初得之时，元气未虚，必推荡之，此通因通用之法。（《丹溪心法》卷一）

> （痢疾……初患的时候，元气没有亏虚，应该用泻下疏通的方法治疗，这就是"通因通用"的治法。）

In terms of dysentery… at its onset, original qi is not deficient so purgative method should be used, which is treating the flowing by promoting flow. (*Danxi's Mastery of Medicine*)

塞因塞用

Treating the Blocked by Blocking

反治法之一。用补益药物治疗具有闭塞不通症状的虚性病证的治法。此法适用于脏腑气血阴阳不足，功能低下所致的闭塞不通之证。如精气不足，冲任亏损的闭经，治当填补下元，滋养肝肾，养血益气以调其经。大便虚秘，因于血虚者宜养血润燥；因于气虚传导无力者当益气健脾；阳虚便秘治以温阳；津亏便秘治宜养津补阴，增水行舟。又如小便不利，或因于肺气不足，通调无权；或因于中气下陷，清气不升，浊阴不降；或由于肾阳亏虚，命门火衰，膀胱气化无权；治疗当分别予以补益肺气，复其通调水道之权；或补益中气，使脾气升运，浊阴自降；或温补肾阳，化气行水。

The term refers to one of the paradoxical treatments, meaning treating the deficient pattern with obstructive signs and symptoms by using tonifying medicine. This method is applicable to relieving obstructive patterns due to the hypofunction of zang-fu organs caused by insufficiency of yin, yang, qi, and blood. For example, amenorrhea due to insufficiency of essential qi and deficiency of thoroughfare vessel and conception vessel should be treated by replenishing kidney qi and nourishing the liver, the kidney, and blood to regulate menstruation. In terms of deficient constipation, it requires nourishing blood and moistening dryness in the case of blood deficiency; reinforcing qi to invigorate spleen yang in the case of qi deficiency causing inability to transport essence; warming yang qi in the case of yang deficiency; or nourishing fluids and supplementing yin to promote body-fluid production and bowel movement in the case of fluid deficiency. As for dysuria, it requires supplementing lung qi to restore its regulation of waterway in the case of insufficiency of lung qi causing disorder of regulating water passage; supplementing middle-qi to ascend spleen qi and descend turbid yin in the case of spleen-qi sinking causing failure to ascend the clear and descend the turbid; or warming kidney yang and transforming qi to promote diuresis in the case of kidney-yang deficiency and life-gate-fire decline leading to qi-transformation disorder of the urinary bladder.

【曾经译法】 treat the pseudo-obstructive disease with tonics; TREATING OBSTRUCTION BY TONIFICATION; treating the obstruction-syndrome with tonics; using tonifying method to treat obstructive syndrome; treating the stopped by stopping; treating obstruction by tonification; treating obstructive syndrome with nourishing therapy

【现行译法】 treating obstructive diseases by tonification; filling for the stuffed; using blockage when the cause is blockage; treat stuffiness with tonic; treating the stopped by stopping; treating obstructive syndrome with dredging method; treat block with block

【标准译法】 treating the blocked by blocking

【翻译说明】 "塞因"指闭塞不同的虚症，曾经被译为 obstruction, stagnation 或 blockage。其中，obstruction 常指阻塞道路、门口、通道等，stagnation 常指停滞不前，不发展，萧条等，blockage 表示阻塞，堵塞。考虑到简洁性和回译性，并且体现"塞因塞用"是中医治则之一，与"通因通用"译法相对应，本书倾向于将"塞因塞用"翻译为 treating the blocked by blocking。

引例 Citations:

◎塞因塞用，通因通用，必伏其所主，而先其所因。（《素问·至真要大论》）

（用补益药物治疗虚性闭塞不通的病证，用通利的药物治疗实性通泻的病证。要制伏其主病，必先找出致病的原因。）

Treat the blocked by blocking, and treat the flowing by promoting flow. To cure a disease, the cause must be made clear first. (*Plain Conversation*)

◎塞因塞用者，如下气虚乏，中焦气壅，欲散满则更虚其下……峻补其下则下自实，中满自除矣。（《内经知要》卷下）

> （塞因塞用者，例如下焦正气亏虚，中焦之气壅滞，想行气消除胀满，则使下焦正气更加亏虚……强力补益下焦正气，则下焦正气恢复，中焦胀满自然可以消除。）

Treat the blocked by blocking. For example, when healthy qi in the lower energizer is deficient and that in the middle energizer stagnates, promoting the flow of qi to relieve abdominal distension may worsen the deficiency of healthy qi in the lower energizer... Instead, greatly reinforcing healthy qi in the lower energizer can help with qi restoration, which relieves distension and fullness in the middle energizer. (*Essentials of the Internal Canon of Medicine*)

标本缓急

Branch, Root, the Non-acute, and the Acute

针对复杂多变的病证中各种因素区分主次、本末、轻重、缓急，并分析其关系之演变，以确定治疗措施的思维方法。标与本，本义分别指草木的末梢与根干，可引申为主与次的关系。所以，标与本作为相对的概念，在不同场合，可以有不同的具体含义。就疾病过程中的正与邪而言，则正气为本，邪气为标；就病因与症状而言，则病因为本，症状为标；就发病之先后而言，则先病、原发病为本，后病、继发病为标；从病变部位来说，则内部脏腑为本，外部体表是标。在复杂的病证中，运用标本理论找出主要矛盾或矛盾的主要方面，分清主次关系，区别轻重缓急加以施治，一般病症急重时，标急则先治其标，本急宜先治其本，标本俱急应标本同治；病症缓和时，先治其本或标本兼顾。

The term refers to the way of thinking that appropriate therapeutic methods should be determined based on the differentiation of primary factors and secondary factors, the branch and the root, the minor and the major, as well as the non-acute and the acute and on the analysis of their relationships among the various factors in complicated and variable patterns. *Biao* and *ben*, literally referring to the branch and the root of a plant, can be figuratively used to explain the relationship between the primary and the secondary factors. Therefore, as a pair of contrary concepts, they have multiple connotations in different contexts. For example, with respect to healthy qi (root), pathogenic qi is regarded as the branch in the disease development. In the relation between disease cause and symptoms, the former is the root, and the latter is the branch. In terms of disease sequence, the old or primary disease is the root and the new or secondary disease is the branch. Finally, as for diseased sites, the internal zang-fu organs are viewed as the roots and the exterior manifestations are the branches. In terms of treating complex patterns, it is advisable to identify the primary conflict or the primary aspect of the conflict, distinguishing the primary from the secondary, the major from the minor, as well as the acute from the non-acute to cure diseases. Generally, in acute and severe cases, either the branch or the root should be treated first if it is acute; if both are acute, they should be treated at the same time. In non-acute cases, the root should be treated first or both the root and the branch are treated at the same time.

【曾经译法】/

【现行译法】/

【标准译法】branch, root, the non-acute, and the acute

【翻译说明】"标本"的曾经译法包括 primary and secondary, principal and subordinate aspects, biao and ben, symptoms and root cause, branch and root 等，其中 branch and root 比较常用。考虑到简洁性和回译性，将"标本缓急"译为 branch, root, the non-acute, and the acute。

引例 Citations:

◎医不明标本缓急，误人性命，固所不免矣。(《时病论》卷一)

（医生不明白标本缓急的道理，贻害人的生命，确实是难以避免的。）

If the doctors did not know the principle of the branch and the root as well as that of the non-acute and the acute, it is inevitable to misdiagnose the diseases and bring harm to patients. (*Treatise on Seasonal Diseases*)

◎病症错乱，当分标本，相其缓急而施治法。(《医学心悟》卷一)

（病症复杂，应当区分标本，观察病症的缓急而采用相应的治法。）

If the disease is complicated, one should differentiate between the root and the branch as well as the non-acute and the acute before giving corresponding treatment. (*Medical Understanding*)

◎至于既传之后，则标本缓急，先后分合，用药必两处兼顾，而又不杂不乱，则诸病亦可渐次平复。(《医学源流论》卷上)

（至于疾病已经传变之后，就要分清标本缓急，治疗的先后以及单独或同时治疗，用药必须标本兼顾，有序而不杂乱，这样各种疾病就可以逐渐平复。）

In the case of disease transformation, it is advisable to differentiate between the branch and the root as well as the non-acute and the acute. The treatment sequence and whether to treat one disease only or two or more simultaneously should be made clear. Medicinals for treating both the root cause and symptoms (the branch) should be used. If things are dealt with in order, various diseases can be relieved. (*Treatise on the Origin and Development of Medicine*)

扶正祛邪

Reinforcing Healthy Qi and Eliminating Pathogenic Qi

中医治疗疾病的基本法则之一，即扶助正气，祛除邪气。扶正，指扶助正气，增强体质，提高机体抗邪和康复能力的治疗法则，包括益气、养血、滋阴、温阳、填精，以及补益脏腑之法等，适用于正气亏虚的各种虚性病理变化。祛邪，指祛除病邪，消解内生有害之物，抑制亢奋的病理反应，减少病理损伤的治疗法则，包括发汗、涌吐、攻下、清热、消导、祛风、利湿、化痰、活血化瘀等，适用于邪气盛实的各种实性病理变化。扶正与祛邪两者相互为用，相辅相成，扶正增强了正气，有助于机体祛除病邪，即所谓"正胜邪自去"；祛邪则在邪气被祛的同时，减免了对正气的侵害，即所谓"邪去正自安"。

The term refers to one of the fundamental therapeutic principles in traditional Chinese medicine. Reinforcing healthy qi means improving the anti-pathogenic ability and promoting rehabilitation by supporting healthy qi and enhancing body constitution, including various methods such as boosting qi, nourishing blood, enriching yin, warming yang, supplementing essence, and fortifying the zang-fu organs, etc. It is applicable to the treatment of various deficiency patterns caused by deficient healthy qi. Eliminating pathogenic qi means inhibiting hyperactive pathological reactions and reducing pathological damage by eliminating pathogenic factors and resolving internally-generated harmful things, including methods such as promoting sweat, inducing vomiting, purgation, clearing heat, relieving food stagnation, dispelling wind, draining dampness, resolving phlegm, and invigorating blood to dissolve stasis, etc. It is applicable to the treatment of various excess patterns caused by excessive pathogenic qi. Reinforcing healthy qi and eliminating pathogenic qi are opposite but complementary methods, forming an interdependent relationship. When healthy qi is enhanced, it will assist the body to expel pathogenic qi, which is described as "with strengthened healthy qi, pathogenic qi will recede automatically." On the other hand, when pathogenic qi is eliminated, healthy qi will be protected from further impairment, which is described as "with pathogenic qi being dispelled, healthy qi is safeguarded naturally."

【曾经译法】 support the healthy energy and eliminate the evil factors; REINFORCING BODY RESISTANCE TO ELIMINATE PATHOGENS; supporting healthy energy to eliminate evils; strengthening the genuine-qi to eliminate the evil-qi

【现行译法】 supporting the body resistance (扶正); supporting vital qi (扶正); supporting the healthy and eliminating the evil; strengthening healthy qi to eliminate pathogenic factors; reinforcing the healthy qi to eliminate pathogenic qi; reinforce the healthy and eliminate the pathogenic; strengthening vital qi to eliminate pathogenic factor

【标准译法】 reinforcing healthy qi and eliminating pathogenic qi

【翻译说明】 "正""邪"采用常用译法，分别译为 healthy qi 和 pathogenic qi。译词 reinforce 强调通过额外补充物质材料或助力达到增强的目的，符合中医"扶正"的语境。译词 eliminate 强调彻底去除、摆脱某物，符合中医"祛邪"的语境。"扶正"与"祛邪"可分别作为治则单独使用，二者并用则相辅相成，因此用 and 表并列为妥。

引例 Citations:

◎奠阴承气之法，又为扶正祛邪之要着也。(《疫喉浅论》卷下)

（滋补阴液，承气汤攻下的治法，就又成了扶正祛邪的首要之事。）

The therapeutic method of combining yin-fluid nourishment and purging with *Chengqi* Decoction (Decoction for Purging Disestive Qi), is an important example of reinforcing healthy qi and eliminating pathogenic qi. (*The Simple Treatise on Seasonal Throat Disorders*)

◎治虚邪者，当先顾正气，正气存则不致于害，且补中自有攻意……治实证者，当去其邪，邪去则身安。(《张氏医通》卷二)

>（治疗正气虚而邪气不盛的病证，应当先补益正气，正气恢复则邪气不至于进一步损害人体，这就是补益之中而有祛邪之意……治疗邪气盛而正气不虚的病证，应当祛除邪气，邪气得以祛除，身体就可以安和。）

Supplementing healthy qi should be given top priority in the treatment of a deficiency pattern (deficiency of healthy qi with mild pathogenic qi). Once healthy qi is restored, pathogenic qi can no longer do further harm to the body. Therefore, the therapy involves dispelling pathogenic qi while supplementing healthy qi... In the treatment of an excess pattern (exuberance of pathogenic qi with no deficiency of healthy qi), expelling pathogenic qi should be prioritized. Once pathogenic qi is removed, health will be automatically restored. (*Comprehensive Medicine by Doctor Zhang Lu*) tiáolǐ yīnyáng

调理阴阳

Regulating Yin and Yang

纠正疾病过程中机体阴阳的偏盛偏衰，损其有余，补其不足，恢复和重建人体的阴阳有序稳态。在中医学中阴阳的含义有属性与本体的区别。就属性角度而言，阴阳的失调可谓是对病变机理的高度概括，可涵盖各种病理情况，如表里出入、寒热转化、邪正盛衰、营卫不和、气血失调等。因此，调理阴阳就成了中医治疗的最高原则，可以涵纳扶正祛邪、调整脏腑、调理气血、调和营卫、协调升降等。就本体阴阳而言，阴阳失调主要是指机体阴阳之间的偏盛、偏衰、互损、格拒、亡失等变化，而其基本病机为偏盛或偏衰。因此，调理阴阳是指针对阴阳盛衰变化的损其有余、补其不足和损益兼用等治则。一般讲调理阴阳多指后者而言。

The term refers to adjusting yin-yang disharmony and re-establishing yin-yang balance by reducing the excess and supplementing the deficiency. In traditional Chinese medicine (TCM), yin and yang can be used as an overarching pair for classification or two entity concepts. As classification standards, imbalance between yin and yang covers and explains various pathological changes, including exterior-interior transmission, cold-heat transformation, predominance or debilitation of healthy qi or pathogenic qi, disharmony between nutrient qi and defense qi, and qi-blood imbalance. Therefore, to regulate yin and yang is regarded as the fundamental principle in TCM therapy, including specific sub-principles such as reinforcing healthy qi and eliminating pathogenic qi, regulating the zang-fu organs, regulating qi and blood, harmonizing nutritive and defensive aspects, as well as promoting regular ascending and descending of qi. When yin and yang are regarded as entity concepts, yin-yang imbalance refers to the abnormal state of yin or yang in the human body, i.e., predominance, debilitation, mutual impairment, repelling, or even loss of yin or yang, among which predominance or debilitation of yin or yang is the primary etiology. Therefore, in this case, to regulate yin and yang generally refers to the therapeutic principles of reducing the excess or supplementing the deficiency in accordance with the changes in the predominance or debilitation of yin or yang, and combining reducing with supplementing methods, which is usually regarded as the common interpretation of this term.

【曾经译法】 regulation of yin and yang (调整阴阳); coordinate Yin and Yang (调和阴阳)

【现行译法】 regulating yin and yang (调整阴阳); regulating yin and yang; coordinating yin and yang; regulate yin and yang

【标准译法】 regulating yin and yang

【翻译说明】 "调理"选用 regulate，即通过规则控制某些活动或过程，符合"调理阴阳"应遵循阴阳转化关系而进行治疗的内涵。yin，yang 为中医"阴""阳"的通用译法。

引例 Citations:

◎此药安心养神，调理阴阳，使无偏胜。(《医学正传》卷一)

（这种药可以安心养神，调理阴阳，使阴阳没有偏胜。）

This formula tranquilizes the mind and nourishes the spirit. It can regulate yin and yang to restore a balance. (*Orthodoxy of Medicine*)

◎故用黄连汤寒温互用，甘苦并施，以调理阴阳而和解之也。(《医宗金鉴》卷五)

（所以用黄连汤寒温互用，甘苦并施，以调理阴阳使其恢复到和谐状态。）

Therefore, *Huanglian* Decoction (Coptis Decoction) is used. With a combination of cold and warm, sweet and bitter medicinals in the formula, yin and yang are regulated to achieve harmony. (*Golden Mirror of Medical Tradition*)

◎十味香薷饮，治内伤不足，调理阴阳，止泄泻。（《医林撮要》卷二）

　　（十味香薷饮，可以治疗内伤引起的虚证，调理阴阳，止泄泻。）

Shiwei Xiangru Drink (Ten-ingredient Molsa Drink) works to treat various deficiency patterns resulting from internal damage. It regulates yin and yang, and relieves diarrhea. (*Summary of Key Medical Formula*)

阴病治阳

Treating Yin Diseases from Yang Aspect

阴相对偏盛出现的虚寒证，治疗通过温补阳气以制约阴的相对偏盛。又称为"温阳散寒"或"益火之源，以消阴翳"(《黄帝内经素问》王冰注)。由于阴阳之间是相互制约的，若阳虚不能制约阴，阴即相对偏盛，就会出现一系列虚寒的征象。因此，对于这种阴的相对偏盛，应当从阳虚的角度进行治疗。

The term means that yang qi should be supplemented to restrict excessive yin in treating deficiency-cold pattern due to relative predominance of yin. It is also known as "warming yang to dissipate cold" or "replenishing the source of fire (yang) to dissipate excessive yin." (*Plain Conversation in Yellow Emperor's Internal Canon of Medicine* Annotated by Wang Bing) Yin and yang restrict each other. When yang is too deficient to restrain yin, yin will become relatively predominant, and various manifestations of deficiency cold may occur. Therefore, in treating the relative predominance of yin, the focus is on the deficient aspect and yang should be supplemented.

【曾经译法】 treat *yang* for *yin* disease; TREATING YANG FOR THE YIN DISEASE; treating yang for yin diseases; treating yin disease from yang aspect; treat Yang for Yin disease

【现行译法】 treating yang for yin disease; treating yang for yin diseases; treating yang to cure yin disease; treating yin disease from yang aspect; yang aspect treated for diseases of the yin nature; yin disease treated through yang

【标准译法】 treating yin diseases from yang aspect

【翻译说明】 "阴病治阳"是指治疗阴偏盛的虚寒证，采用温补阳气之法。译文 treating yin diseases from yang aspect 用介词 from 明确了词语内部逻辑关系，兼具了意合与形合，回译性较好。

引例 Citations:

◎审其阴阳，以别柔刚，阳病治阴，阴病治阳。(《素问·阴阳应象大论》)
    (观察病的在阴在阳，来决定应当用柔剂还是刚剂。病在阳的，
    也可治其阴；病在阴的，也可治其阳。)

By differentiating whether the disease lies in yin or yang aspect, one can decide what formula should be used. Treat a yin disease from yang aspect, and vice versa. (*Plain Conversation*)

◎阴胜者阳伤，治其阳者，补水中之火也。(《内经知要》卷下)
    (阴偏盛是由于阳气损伤，治疗阳就是温补肾阳。)

Relative predominance of yin results from the impairment of yang qi. To treat it, yang qi should be supplemented by warming and tonifying kidney yang. (*Essentials of the Internal Canon of Medicine*) yángbìng zhìyīn

阳病治阴

Treating Yang Diseases from Yin Aspect

阳相对偏盛出现的虚热证，治疗通过滋补阴液以制约阳的相对偏盛，又称为"滋阴清热"或"壮水之主，以制阳光"（《黄帝内经素问》王冰注）。由于阴阳之间是相互制约的，若阴虚不能制约阳，阳即相对偏盛，就会出现一系列虚热的征象。因此，对于这种阳的相对偏盛，应当从阴虚的角度进行治疗。

The term means that yin fluids can be enriched to restrict excessive yang in treating deficiency-heat pattern due to relative predominance of yang. It is also known as "enriching yin fluids to clear heat" or "strengthening the source of water (yin) to restrict hyperactive yang." (*Plain Conversation in Yellow Emperor's Internal Canon of Medicine Annotated by Wang Bing*) Yin and yang restrict each other. When yin is too deficient to restrain yang, yang will become relatively predominant, and various manifestations of deficiency heat may occur. Therefore, in treating relative predominance of yang, the focus is on the deficient aspect and yin should be supplemented.

【曾经译法】 treat *yin* for *yang* disease; treating yin for yang diseases; treating yang disease from yin aspect; treat Yin for Yang disease

【现行译法】 treating yin for the yang disease; treating yin for yang disease; treating yin to cure yang disease; treating yang disease from yin aspect; treating the yin aspect for diseases of yang nature; yang disease treated through yin

【标准译法】 treating yang diseases from yin aspect

【翻译说明】 "阳病治阴"指治疗阳偏盛的虚热证，采用滋补阴液之法。译文 treating yang diseases from yin aspect 用介词 from 明确了词语内部逻辑关系，兼具了意合与形合，回译性较好。

引例 Citations:

◎阳胜者阴伤，治其阴者，补水之主也。（《内经知要》卷下）

（阳偏盛的是由于阴液损伤，治疗阴就是滋补阴液。）

Relative predominance of yang results from the damage of yin fluids. To treat it, yin fluids should be supplemented by nourishing the source of yin. (*Essentials of the Internal Canon of Medicine*)

◎阳胜者阴必病，阴胜者阳必病，如"诸寒之而热者，取之阴，热之而寒者，取之阳"；"壮水之主，以制阳光，益火之源，以消阴翳"之类，皆阳病治阴、阴病治阳之道也。（《医经原旨》卷三）

（阳胜必然引起阴的不足，阴胜必然引起阳的不足，诸如"诸寒之而热者，取之阴，热之而寒者，取之阳"；"壮水之主，以制阳光，益火之源，以消阴翳"之类的治法，都遵循阳病治阴、阴病治阳的规律。）

Yang predominance undoubtedly results in yin deficiency, and vice versa. There are sayings about therapeutic methods as follows: "Treat heat patterns with cold medicinals to purge heat—if heat is unrelieved, treat with yin-nourishing medicinals; treat cold patterns with hot medicinals to dissipate cold—if cold is unrelieved, treat with yang-supplementing medicinals" and "strengthen the source of water to restrict hyperactive yang; replenish the source of fire to dissipate excessive yin." These methods follow the principle of treating yang diseases from yin aspect, and treating yin diseases from yang aspect. (*Original Decrees of Medicine*) yīn zhōng qiú yáng

阴中求阳

Obtaining Yang from Yin

阴中求阳，是指治疗阳偏衰时，在补阳剂中适当佐用滋阴药。由于阴阳之间存在着互根互用的关系，故在治疗阳气偏衰的病证时，组方用药可利用此关系，以补阳为主适当配合补阴药，以促进阳气的化生，如右归丸的组方。

The term refers to the addition of yin-enriching medicinals to the yang-tonifying formula in the treatment of yang debilitation. As yin and yang are mutually dependent and rooted, one can make good use of this relationship in composing a formula for the treatment of yang-qi debilitation to achieve better therapeutic effects: mainly use yang-tonifying medicinals and add a few yin-nourishing ones to facilitate the generation and transformation of yang qi. The composition of *You Gui* Pill (Right-restoring Pill) is a case in point.

【曾经译法】 treat Yang in Yin

【现行译法】 obtaining yang from yin; treat yin for yang; treating yin for yang

【标准译法】 obtaining yang from yin

【翻译说明】 术语重点在于"求阳"，"阴"为方式和来源，因此翻译时适当调整语序，将"求阳"这一目的和结果前置，突出重点。此外，"求"选用 obtain，而非 treat，强调获得、获取之意，同时也与"阴病治阳"中以 treat 翻译"治"相区分。

引例 Citations:

◎故善补阳者，必于阴中求阳，则阳得阴助而生化无穷；善补阴者，必于

阳中求阴，则阴得阳升而泉源不竭。(《景岳全书·新方八阵》)

（所以善补阳者，必于阴中求阳，阳气得到阴气的资助则能不断
化生；善补阴者，必于阳中求阴，阴气得到阳气的资助则产生的
来源充沛。）

Doctors adept at the methods of tonifying yang always obtain yang from yin to ensure continuous generation of yang with the addition of yin. Likewise, those good at the methods of nourishing yin obtain yin from yang to ensure abundant generation of yin with the help of yang. (*Jingyue's Complete Works*)

◎阴中求阳，阳中求阴，盖阴阳互根也。(《理瀹骈文》)

（所以阴中求阳，阳中求阴，是因为阴阳互根互用。）

The rationale for the principles of obtaining yang from yin and obtaining yin from yang is that yin and yang are mutually dependent and rooted. (*Rhymed Discourse on External Remedies*)

阳中求阴

Obtaining Yin from Yang

阳中求阴，是指治疗阴偏衰时，在滋阴剂中适当佐用补阳药。由于阴阳之间存在着互根互用的关系，故在治疗阴精偏衰的病证时，组方用药可利用此关系，以补阴为主适当配合补阳药，以促进阴精的生成，如左归丸的组方。

The term refers to the addition of yang-tonifying medicinals to the yin-enriching formula in the treatment for yin debilitation. As yin and yang are mutually dependent and rooted, one can make good use of this relationship in composing a formula for the treatment of yin-essence debilitation to achieve better therapeutic effects: mainly use yin-nourishing medicinals and add a few yang-tonifying ones to promote the generation and transformation of yin essence. The composition of *Zuo Gui* Pill (Left-restoring Pill) is a case in point.

【曾经译法】 getting yin from yang; treat Yin in Yang

【现行译法】 obtaining yin from yang; treat yang for yin; treating yang for yin

【标准译法】 obtaining yin from yang

【翻译说明】 术语重点在于"求阴"，"阳"为方式和来源，因此翻译时适当调整语序，将"求阴"这一目的和结果前置，突出重点。此外，"求"选用 obtain，而非 treat，强调获得、获取之意，同时也与"阳病治阴"中以 treat 翻译"治"相区分。

引例 Citations:

◎善补阴者，必于阳中求阴，则阴得阳升而泉源不竭。（《景岳全书·新方八阵》）

（善补阴者，必于阳中求阴，阴气得到阳气的资助则产生的来源充沛。）

Doctors good at the methods of enriching yin obtain yin from yang to ensure abundant generation of yin with the help of yang. (*Jingyue's Complete Works*)

◎故经云：故善补阳者于阴中求阳，善补阴者于阳中求阴。（《医理真传》卷三）

（所以《内经》说：善补阳的医生于阴中求阳，善补阴的医生于阳中求阴。）

Therefore, *Yellow Emperor's Internal Canon of Medicine* says that doctors good at the methods of tonifying yang will obtain yang from yin, while those good at the methods of enriching yin usually obtain yin from yang. (*True Transmission of Medical Principles*) yìqiáng fúruò

抑强扶弱

Inhibiting the Strong and Supporting the Weak

根据五行相克规律所确定的基本治疗原则。五行相克异常所表现出的病理变化，虽有相克太过、不及和反克等不同，但发生的原因不外乎强弱两个方面，即一方过强，表现为功能亢进；另一方偏弱，表现为功能衰退。因此，治疗上须同时采取抑强扶弱的手段，或侧重于制其强盛，使弱者易于恢复；或侧重于扶其不足，避免弱者被克或相克病情的进一步发展。抑强，适用于相克太过引起的相乘和相侮，如肝气横逆，乘脾犯胃，出现肝脾不调、肝胃不和等证，称为木旺乘土，治疗应以疏肝、平肝为主。扶弱，适用于相克不及引起的相乘和相侮，如脾胃虚弱，肝气乘虚犯脾，导致肝脾不和之证，称为土虚木乘，治疗当以健脾益气为主。

The term refers to a primary therapeutic principle developed in accordance with the restraining cycle among the five elements. Although abnormal restraining relationships may vary in forms including excess, inadequacy, and counter restraining, the causes fall into two broad categories—the strong and the weak. When an element is excessively strong, it will manifest signs of hyperfunction. By contrast, hypofunction occurs when one gets excessively weak. Therefore, in treatment, the principle of inhibiting the strong and supporting the weak should be carried out simultaneously, emphasizing either inhibiting the strong to help the weak restore to normal, or supporting the weak to avoid being restricted or further aggravation. On the one hand, the principle of inhibiting the strong is applicable to over-restriction or counter-restriction due to excessive restricting. For example, excessive liver (wood) qi over-restricts the spleen and stomach (earth), leading to liver-spleen or liver-stomach disharmony, which is described as excessive wood (liver) over-restricting earth (spleen) and should be treated chiefly by soothing and pacifying liver qi. On the other hand, the principle of supporting the weak is applicable to over-restriction or counter-restriction due to the insufficiency of restriction, such as liver (wood) qi attacking deficient spleen (earth) leading to liver-spleen disharmony, which is described as earth (spleen) deficiency leading to over-restriction by wood (liver) and should be treated chiefly by fortifying spleen qi.

【曾经译法】 /

【现行译法】 inhibiting the strong and supporting the weak; inhibiting excessiveness (抑强); supporting weakness (扶弱)

【标准译法】 inhibiting the strong and supporting the weak

【翻译说明】 "抑强扶弱" 包含一 "抑" 一 "扶"，一 "强" 一 "弱"，两组词互为反义，应分别对应参照翻译。"抑" 选用 inhibit，即阻止、阻碍之意; "扶" 选用 support，即支持、帮助之意。译词 the strong 和 the weak 既对应 "强" "弱" 的抽象表达，又较为简短。

引例 Citations:

◎五气有偏胜，脏腑刚柔不同，用药以抑强扶弱，取中而治。(《医经小学》)

（五行之气有偏胜，脏腑有刚柔不同，用药应当抑强扶弱，以达到平衡。）

Five climatic qi may vary in intensity, and zang-fu organs vary from tenderness to resolution. Therefore, in treatment, the strong should be inhibited and the weak supported so that qi can be regulated to achieve balance. (*Elementary Learning of Medical Canons*)

◎又须审二经五行之气，抑强扶弱，以致和气。(《伤寒论集注》卷九)

（又必须审察阳明、少阳经及五脏之气的盛衰，抑强扶弱，而使气得以调和。）

Besides, the conditions of *yangming* and *shaoyang* meridians as well as the five zang-organs should be carefully observed regarding predominance and debilitation. By inhibiting the strong and supporting the weak, a harmonious state of qi can be achieved. (*Collected Commentaries on "Treatise on Cold Damage"*)

抑木扶土

Inhibiting Wood to Support Earth

用疏肝健脾或平肝和胃的药物来治疗肝脾不和或肝气犯胃证的方法。故又称之为疏肝健脾法、平肝和胃法、调理肝脾法、调和肝胃法。根据五行与脏腑配属关系，肝属木，脾胃属土。抑木扶土，即抑制肝气的偏盛而扶助脾胃的不足。临床常用于木旺乘土，木不疏土的肝脾不和、肝胃不和证，代表方如逍遥散、痛泻要方等。

The term refers to the therapeutic method of treating liver-spleen disharmony by soothing the liver and fortifying the spleen or relieving liver qi attacking the stomach by pacifying liver qi and harmonizing the stomach. It is also known as soothing the liver and fortifying the spleen, or pacifying liver qi and harmonizing the stomach, or regulating the liver and the spleen, or harmonizing the liver and the stomach. According to the correspondence between the five elements and the zang-fu organs, the liver pertains to wood; the spleen and the stomach pertain to earth. Therefore, this term refers to suppressing the hyperactive liver qi to strengthen the deficient spleen-stomach qi. Clinically, this method is used to treat liver-spleen or liver-stomach disharmony due to hyperactive liver (wood) qi over-restricting the spleen and stomach (earth), or stagnated liver (wood) qi failing to regulate the qi flow of the spleen and stomach (earth). Representative formulas include *Xiaoyao* Powder (Free Wanderer Powder) and *Tongxie Yaofang* (Important Formula for Painful Diarrhea).

【曾经译法】 /

【现行译法】 /

【标准译法】 inhibiting wood to support earth

【翻译说明】 "抑""扶"的选词与前词"抑强扶弱"保持一致，"木""土"均采用五行元素译法，以保留此中医治则术语的特色，同时使英译术语较为简短精炼。"肝郁"为基本病机，肝郁导致脾胃气机运行受阻，因此应为"抑木"以"扶土"，为递进关系。

引例 Citations:

◎肝木太强，则脾土受制……小建中汤之义，全在抑木扶土。(《医方论》卷三)

（肝气偏盛，则会制约脾土……小建中汤的方义，全在于抑木扶土。）

If liver (wood) qi is hyperactive, it will over-restrict spleen (earth) qi... The rationale behind *Xiao Jianzhong* Decoction (Minor Center-fortifying Decoction) is based on the principle of inhibiting wood to support earth. (*Treatise on Medical Formulas*)

◎土既受伤，木安有不侮之理，抑木扶土，此症急治之法。(《徐氏四世医案合编》)

（脾土既然已经受损，哪有肝气不来相侮的道理，抑木扶土，是迅速治疗这种病症的方法。）

With the impairment of spleen qi, how can the liver wood not over-restrict the spleen earth? Therefore, the suitable method to promptly address this disorder is inhibiting wood to support earth. (*Collected Medical Case Records by Doctor Xu in Four Generations*)

佐金平木

Supporting Metal to Suppress Wood

用清肃肺气的药物以抑制肝木，又称为清泻肝肺法。根据五行与脏腑配属关系，肺属金，肝属木。佐金平木，辅佐肺气的肃降，平抑肝气的偏盛，临床多用于肝火偏盛，影响肺气清肃之证，常见两胁窜痛，气喘不平，脉弦等症，药物多用吴茱萸、炒桑白皮、苏梗、枇杷叶等，使肺气下降，肝气舒畅。

The term, also known as clearing liver and lung fire, refers to the therapeutic method of suppressing hyperactive liver (wood) qi by directing lung (metal) qi downward. According to the correspondence between the five elements and the zang-fu organs, the lung pertains to metal, and the liver pertains to wood. Supporting metal to suppress wood involves aiding lung qi to descend to relieve the excess of liver qi. Clinically, this method is used to treat hyperactive liver fire affecting the lung's function in purification, manifested as wandering pain in the hypochondrium, panting, and a wiry pulse, etc. Medicinals such as *wuzhuyu* (*Fructus Evodiae*, medicinal evodia fruit), dry-fried *sangbaipi* (*Cortex Mori*, white mulberry root-bark), *sugeng* (*Caulis Perillae*, perilla stem), and *pipaye* (*Folium Eriobotryae*, loquat leaf) are often used to direct lung qi downward to soothe liver qi.

【曾经译法】 support the metal (lung) to calm the wood (liver); CALMING THE WOOD BY CLEARING THE METAL; supporting metal to suppress wood; treating the metal to subdue the wood

【现行译法】 treating the lung (metal) to subdue hyperactivity of the liver (wood); supporting metal to suppress wood; supporting lung to suppress liver

【标准译法】 supporting metal to suppress wood

【翻译说明】 "佐"被译为 treat 或 support，"佐"意为佐助、辅助。译词

treat 为广义的治疗之意，过于宽泛，不够准确，因此 support
较为合适。"平"被译为 subdue 或 suppress，二词均有压抑、
克制之意。"平木"实为抑木，选用 suppress，因其含有抑制
生理功能、生长的含义，与"木"意象的搭配更为符合。术
语"佐金平木"的内部逻辑关系为"佐金"从而"平木"，
因此，译为 supporting metal to suppress wood。

引例 Citations:

◎左金丸，佐金平木之义，泻肝火，行湿，为热甚之反佐。(《医学六
要·胁痛门》)

（左金丸，即佐金平木之义，清泻肝火，行湿，为热甚反佐的方
药。）

The name of *Zuo Jin* Pill (Left Metal Pill) suggests its function, i.e., supporting
metal to suppress wood. Specifically, the formula is used to clear liver fire
and drain dampness. With certain hot-natured medicinals as the paradoxical
assistant in the formula, it works to treat extreme heat pattern. (*Six Essentials of
Medicine*)

◎建中汤证……倍芍药泻火除烦，任生姜佐金平木。(《伤寒来苏集》
卷三)

（建中汤证……将芍药用量加倍以泻火除烦，用生姜以佐金
平木。）

To treat the pattern by *Jianzhong* Decoction (Center-fortifying Decoction)…
double the dosage of *shaoyao* (*Radix Paeoniae Alba seu Rubra*, white or red
peony root) to clear fire and relieve vexation, and use *shengjiang* (*Rhizoma
Zingiberis Recens*, fresh ginger) to support metal to suppress wood. (*Collected
Writings on the Renewal of "Treatise on Cold Damage"*)

◎三之气，木邪内肆，加紫菀佐金平木。(《世补斋医书》卷九)

（少阳相火之气，肝木邪气在内肆虐，加紫菀以佐金平木。）

When *shaoyang* qi is dominant, liver (wood) qi tends to be predominant internally, so *ziwan* (*Radix et Rhizoma Asteris*, tatarian aster root) should be added to support the lung metal to suppress the liver wood. (*Medical Works from the Shibu House*) xiènán bǔběi

泻南补北

Purging South and Nourishing North

泻心火补肾水以治疗心肾不交病证的方法，又称为泻火补水法、滋阴降火法、交通心肾法。根据五行与脏腑、方位配属关系，心主火，火属南方；肾主水，水属北方，故称本法为泻南补北法。临床适用于肾阴不足，心火偏旺，水火不济，心肾不交之证。由于泻火之品，多苦寒而燥，有伤津耗液之弊，单用苦寒药则水愈亏。反之，单用甘寒育阴药则又不能扑灭火炎之势，唯有泻火育阴法合用，方可收火折水生之效，代表方如黄连阿胶汤等。

The term refers to the therapeutic method of treating heart-kidney disharmony by reducing heart fire and supplementing kidney water. It is also known as clearing fire and enriching water, or enriching yin and reducing fire, or restoring coordination between the heart and the kidney. According to the correspondence between the five elements and zang-fu organs, and the five element and directions, the heart corresponds to fire, which pertains to south and the kidney corresponds to water, which pertains to north, hence the term "purging south and nourishing north." Clinically, this method is applicable to heart-kidney (fire-water) disharmony due to insufficient kidney yin and effulgent heart fire. Fire-clearing medicinals, usually bitter, cold and dry, tend to damage fluids; if used alone, they will result in severer fluid damage. Yin-nourishing medicinals, mostly bitter and cold, if used alone, cannot restrict the fire from flaming upward. Therefore, only by combining fire-clearing and yin-nourishing methods can the effect of restraining fire and generating water be achieved. *Huanglian Ejiao* Decoction (Coptis and Donkey-hide Gelatin Decoction) stands as a representative formula.

【曾经译法】 purging the south and tonifying the north

【现行译法】 reducing the south while reinforcing the north; purging south and nourishing north; purging heart-fire and nourishing kidney-water

【标准译法】 purging south and nourishing north

【翻译说明】 "泻南补北"中"泻南"实为泻心火之意，"泻"被译为 reduce 或 purge，其中 reduce 泛指减少、降低，而 purge 经常表示净化、清洗和通便的意思，较为符合"泻火"之意。"补北"实为滋补肾阴，"补"被译为 reinforce 或 nourish，其中 reinforce 泛指加强、强化，而 nourish 具体指滋养、濡养，因此采用 nourish 较为合适。"南""北"是以方位指代心、肾二脏，直译更能体现中医术语特色。"泻南补北"是指既泻心火，又补肾水，二者相辅相成，因此用 and 表示并列。

引例 Citations:

◎舌黑而干者，津枯火炽，急急泻南补北。（《外感温热篇》）

（舌质黑而干燥者，津液枯竭，火热内炽，急用泻南补北法治疗。）

The black and dry tongue body indicates fluid exhaustion with internal blazing fire in a patient. The method of purging south and nourishing north should be adopted promptly. (*Treatment of Externally Contracted Warm Febrile Diseases*)

◎滋阴降火，泻南补北，是知母之长技也。（《本草汇言》卷一）

（滋阴降火，泻南补北，是知母最擅长的。）

To enrich yin and reduce fire or to purge south and nourish north is what *zhimu* (*Rhizoma Anemarrhenae*, common anemarrhena rhizome) excels at. (*Treasury of Words on Materia Medica*)

◎急当滋其化源，泻南补北，壮水制火，则肝木自平，胎气可安。(《女科经纶》卷四)

（应当迅速滋养其源头，采用泻南补北，滋阴降火，这样肝气就平和了，胎气就安稳了。）

Promptly enrich the source of yin by purging south (fire) and nourishing north (water) to pacify liver qi so that fetal qi can be tranquilized. (*Profound Scholarship in Gynecology*) péitǔ zhìshuǐ

培土制水

Banking Up Earth to Restrain Water

温运脾阳或温肾健脾以治疗水湿停聚病证的方法，又称为敦土利水法、健脾利水法、健脾祛湿法等。这里的土，即指脾脏，脾在五行属土；水，是指水湿邪气。临床适用于脾的阳气亏虚，不能运化水湿，使水湿泛滥所致水肿胀满之类的病证，代表方如实脾饮、防己黄芪汤等。

The term refers to the therapeutic method of treating internal accumulation of water and dampness by warming spleen yang or warming the kidney to fortify the spleen. It is also known as the method of regulating earth to remove water, fortifying spleen yang to drain water, or fortifying spleen yang to dispel dampness. According to the correspondence between the five elements and the zang-fu organs, earth refers to the spleen. The word "water" in the term refers to the pathological water or dampness. Clinically, this method is applicable to various disorders manifested as edema, distension, and the feeling of fullness which are due to the overflow of water or dampness as a result of deficient spleen yang failing to transport and transform water normally. Representative formulas include *Shipi* Drink (Spleen-fortifying Drink) and *Fangji Huangqi* Decoction (Stephania Root and Astragalus Decoction).

【曾经译法】 banking up earth (培土); strengthen Earth to control Water

【现行译法】 tonifying the spleen (earth) to restrain water; banking up earth (培土); banking up earth to control water; supplementing spleen to control bladder

【标准译法】 banking up earth to restrain water

【翻译说明】 "培土制水"中"培"被译为bank up，strengthen，tonify，supplement等。"培"为"补"用于形容强健脾胃（土）的具体形象，翻译为bank up能生动地保留原意象。土"制"水，

"制"为五行相克元素之间的制约关系，选用 restrain，以区别"克"的译文 restrict。术语"培土制水"的内部逻辑关系为"培土"以"制水"，因此译为 banking up earth to restrain water。

引例 Citations:

◎桂枝去桂加茯苓白术汤……佐甘、枣有培土制水之功。(《伤寒来苏集》卷一)

（桂枝去桂加茯苓白术汤……配伍甘草、大枣有培土制水的功效。）

Use *Guizhi* Decoction (Cinnamon Twig Decoction) without *guizhi* (*Ramulus Cinnamomi*, Cinnamon Twig) but add in *fuling* (*Poria*, poria) and *baizhu* (*Rhizoma Atractylodis Macrocephalae*, white atractylodes rhizome)... in combination with *gancao* (*Radix et Rhizoma Glycyrrhizae*, licorice root) and *dazao* (*Fructus Jujubae*, Chinese date) to achieve the effect of banking up earth to restrain water. (*Collected Writings on the Renewal of "Treatise on Cold Damage"*)

◎茯苓桂枝甘草大枣汤……桂枝保心气，茯苓泄肾邪，甘草、大枣培土制水。(《伤寒寻源》下集)

（茯苓桂枝甘草大枣汤……桂枝可以保心气，茯苓可以泄肾邪，甘草、大枣的作用是培土制水。）

In *Fuling Guizhi Gancao Dazao* Decoction (Poria, Cinnamon Twig, Licorice Root, and Chinese Date Decoction)... *guizhi* (*Ramulus Cinnamomi*, Cinnamon Twig) consolidates heart qi, *fuling* (*Poria*, poria) discharges pathogenic kidney qi (water), while *gancao* (*Radix et Rhizoma Glycyrrhizae*, licorice root) and *dazao* (*Fructus Jujubae*, Chinese date) work collaboratively to bank up earth to restrain water. (*Seeking Root Causes of Cold Damage*)

◎姜可以宣达阳气，术可以培土制水。(《重编张仲景伤寒论证治发明溯源集》卷四)

(生姜可以宣达阳气，白术可以培土制水。)

Shengjiang (*Rhizoma Zingiberis Recens*, fresh ginger) diffuses yang qi, while *baizhu* (*Rhizoma Atractylodis Macrocephalae*, white atractylodes rhizome) banks up earth to restrain water. (*Revised Collection of Patterns and Treatments Dated Back to Zhang Zhongjing's "Treatise on Cold Damage"*) bǔmǔ xièzǐ

补母泻子

Tonifying Mother Organ and Reducing Child Organ

　　补益母脏而攻泻子脏，是根据五行相生规律所确定的基本治疗原则。按照五行相生规律，五脏之间具有母子关系，生我者为母脏，我生者为子脏。补母，是指一脏的虚证，不仅须补益本脏之虚损，同时还可依据五行递相资生的次序，补益其母脏，通过"相生"作用促使其康复。如肝血不足，除须用补肝血药物外，还可以用补肾益精的方法，通过"水生木"的作用促使肝血恢复。泻子，是指一脏的实证，不仅须泻除本脏之实邪，同时还可依据五行相生的次序，通过泻其子脏，以促进母脏实邪的祛除。如肝火炽盛，除须用清泻肝火的药物外，还可用泻心火的方法消除过旺的肝火。

The term refers to a primary therapeutic principle developed in accordance with the generating cycle among the five elements. According to the mutual-generating principle among the five elements, there exists mother-child relationship among the five zang-organs. The element of "generating" is named as mother organ while that of "being generated" is child organ. Tonifying mother organ suggests that when a zang-organ is in deficiency, apart from supplementing the organ itself, its mother organ could also be strengthened to promote recovery. For example, in the case of liver-blood deficiency, in addition to nourishing the blood of the liver (wood, child organ), the essence of the kidney (water, mother organ) could also be replenished to promote the generation of liver blood. On the other hand, reducing child organ suggests that when a zang-organ is in excess, apart from dispelling the excess pathogenic factors related to the organ itself, its child organ could also be reduced to achieve better effects. For example, with excessive liver fire, in addition to clearing fire of the liver (wood, mother organ), the fire of the heart (fire, child organ) could also be purged to facilitate the elimination of hyperactive liver fire.

【曾经译法】 The Combination of Reinforcing Mother Point and Reducing Son Point (补母泻子法)

【现行译法】 mother-tonifying child-reducing method (补母泻子法)

【标准译法】 tonifying mother organ and reducing child organ

【翻译说明】 "补母泻子"中"补"被译为 reinforce 或 tonify，"泻"被译为 reduce。由于该术语中"补""泻"对象均为泛指的脏腑，故 tonify 和 reduce 较妥。"补母"与"泻子"是在临床可分别独立使用的治法，习惯合称，因此应用 and 表示并列关系。

引例 Citations:

◎虚则补其母，实则泻其子。(《难经·六十九难》)。

（对某脏的虚证，可以采用补其母脏的方法进行治疗；对某脏的实证，可以采用泻其子脏的方法进行治疗。）

To treat the deficiency pattern of a child organ, one could tonify its mother organ. To treat the excess pattern of a mother organ, one could reduce its child organ. (*Canon of Difficult Issues*)

◎以胃居中焦，分行津液于各脏，补胃泻肺，有补母泻子之义也。(《绛雪园古方》卷二)

（因为胃居于中焦，将津液分别输送到各脏，补胃泻肺，有补母泻子的含义。）

The stomach is situated in the middle energizer and distributes body fluids to all other organs. Tonifying the stomach to reduce lung heat therefore follows the rule of tonifying mother organ and reducing child organ. (*Ancient Formulas from the Crimson Snow Garden*)

◎古人补母泻子之法，殆起于此。如肺气既虚，而又有风热或痰饮之实邪，此宜补脾而攻肺，不得补肺与攻肺并用也。（《读医随笔》卷四）

（古人补母泻子的治法，大致起源于此。如肺气既虚，而又有风热或痰饮之实邪，这时应当补脾而攻肺，不可以补肺与攻肺并用。）

The therapeutic method of tonifying mother organ and reducing child organ used by ancient people is perhaps derived from it. For example, if a patient initially has lung-qi deficiency and then is affected by excess pathogenic qi such as wind-heat or phlegm-rheum, one should tonify the spleen and dispel pathogenic qi in the lung instead of simultaneously reinforcing and reducing the lung. (*Random Notes While Reading About Medicine*) péitǔ shēngjīn

培土生金

Banking Up Earth to Generate Metal

通过补益脾气以养肺气的治疗方法，又称为补脾益肺法、补益肺脾法。根据五行与脏腑配属关系，脾属土，肺属金，二者为母子相生关系。考虑到母能令子强壮，故培土生金，即通过培补脾土以促进肺金功能的康复。临床适用于脾气虚弱，生气无源而致肺气虚衰，或因肺气虚而引起的肺脾两虚证，代表方如参苓白术散等。

The term refers to the therapeutic method of nourishing lung qi by tonifying spleen qi, which is also known as the method of replenishing lung qi by tonifying spleen qi. According to the correspondence between the five elements and the zang-fu organs, the spleen corresponds to earth, and the lung corresponds to metal. Due to the mother-child relationship between them, banking up earth (mother, spleen) can help restore the functions of metal (child, lung). Clinically, this method is used to treat lung-qi deficiency due to the lack of generating source because of spleen-qi deficiency, or to treat qi deficiency of both the lung and the spleen as a result of initial lung-qi deficiency. A representative formula is *Shen Ling Baizhu* Power (Ginseng, Poria, and White Atractylodes Powder).

【曾经译法】 earth up to generate metal (strengthen the spleen to benefit the lung); TONIFYING THE SPLEEN TO HELP THE LUNGS; building up the "earth" to supplement the "metal"; banking up earth to generate metal; strengthen Lung (Metal) by way of reinforcing Spleen (Earth)

【现行译法】 reinforcing the spleen (earth) to strengthen the lung (metal); banking up earth to benefit metal; banking up earth to generate metal; supplementing spleen to strengthen lung; building up earth (spleen) to generate metal (lung)

【标准译法】banking up earth to generate metal

【翻译说明】术语中的"培"字被译为 earth up, build up, bank up, reinforce, strengthen, tonify, supplement 等。"培"为"补"用于形容强健脾胃（土）的具体形象，前三个词组能生动地保留原意象，其中 bank up 更为常用，其他词语只能笼统表达增补之意。土"生"金，"生"为五行相克元素之间的相生关系，应借用五行相生的常用英译选词 generate。"培土生金"的内部逻辑关系为"培土"以"生金"，因此译为 banking up earth to generate metal。

引例 Citations:

◎若脾胃虚弱，宜参用培土生金之法。（《医方论》卷一）

（若脾胃虚弱，应当配合使用培土生金的治法。）

If the spleen and the stomach are in deficiency, the therapeutic method of banking up earth to generate metal should be used in combination. (*Treatise on Medical Formulas*)

◎或言滋水清金，或言培土生金，以实为虚，自谓治本。（《医悟》卷五）

（有的人说滋水清金，有的人说培土生金，把实证当作虚证，自称是治本。）

Some suggest enriching water to clear metal. Others advise banking up earth to generate metal. They all think they treat the root cause of the disease. However, neither method is suitable because the disorder indicates an excess pattern instead of a deficiency one. (*Medical Understanding*)

◎再以甘凉培土生金，调理一月，强健如故。（《外证医案汇编》卷四）

（然后用甘凉的药物培土生金，调理一个月，身体强健如平常。）

Then, use sweet and cool medicinals to bank up earth to generate metal. In this way, a strong and healthy state will be restored in one month. (*Collection of Case Records in External Patterns*) zīshuǐ hánmù

滋水涵木

Enriching Water to Moisten Wood

通过滋补肾阴以养肝阴的治疗方法，又称为滋肾养肝法、滋补肝肾法。根据五行与脏腑配属关系，肾属水，肝属木，二者为母子相生关系。当肾阴虚损累及肝脏，导致肝肾阴虚，这一病理转归，谓之水不涵木。治疗时运用滋肾阴以达到润养肝阴，降火潜阳。临床适用于肾阴亏损而肝阴不足，甚或肝火有余、肝阳上亢之证，代表方如大补阴丸、知柏地黄丸、杞菊地黄丸等。

The term refers to the therapeutic method of nourishing liver yin by enriching kidney yin, which is also known as the method of nourishing the liver by supplementing the kidney, or enriching and tonifying both the liver and the kidney. According to the correspondence between the five elements and the zang-fu organs, the kidney corresponds to water and the liver corresponds to wood. As water generates wood, there is a mother-child relationship between the kidney and the liver. When the liver is affected by kidney-yin deficiency and causes yin deficiency of both the liver and the kidney, it is described as kidney water failing to moisten liver wood. To treat it, kidney yin should be supplemented to nourish liver yin to subdue liver fire and suppress hyperactive liver yang. Clinically, this method is applicable to the treatment of various liver disorders resulting from kidney-yin deficiency, for example, liver-yin insufficiency, or even liver-fire superabundance and liver-yang hyperactivity. Representative formulas include *Da Buyin* Pill (Major Yin-supplementing Pill), *Zhi Bai Dihuang* Pill (Anemarrhena, Phellodendron, and Rehmannia Pill) and *Qi Ju Dihuang* Pill (Lycium Berry, Chrysanthemum, and Rehmannia Pill).

【曾经译法】 providing water for the growth of wood; enriching water to nourish wood; replenish Kidney Yin to nourish Liver

【现行译法】 providing water for growth of wood; nourishing the liver and kidney; enriching water to nourish wood; enrich water to moisten wood; nourishing water to moisten wood

【标准译法】enriching water to moisten wood

【翻译说明】术语中的"滋"字被译为 provide, enrich, replenish 或 nourish, "涵"被译为 nourish 或 moisten。"滋""涵"均为"补"用于形容滋养水（肾）、木（肝）之阴的具体形象，翻译时应尽量保留原意象，同时使之与对应脏腑的功能相匹配，分别译为 enrich 和 moisten 较妥。译词 replenish 常对应翻译"益"，nourish 常对应翻译"养"。"滋水涵木"的内部逻辑关系为"滋水"以"涵木"，因此译为 enriching water to moisten wood。

引例 Citations:

◎议以滋水涵木，和阳息风。方用炙甘草、党参、熟地、麦冬、阿胶、芝麻、茯神、枣仁、五味子、牡蛎、小麦、南枣。(《杏轩医案》卷三)

（拟用滋水涵木，和阳息风的治法。药用炙甘草、党参、熟地、麦冬、阿胶、芝麻、茯神、酸枣仁、五味子、牡蛎、浮小麦、南枣。）

The therapeutic method of enriching water to moisten wood is used to pacify liver yang to extinguish wind. The formula is composed of *zhigancao* (*Radix et Rhizoma Glycyrrhizae Praeparata cum Melle*, prepared licorice root), *dangshen* (*Radix Codonopsis*, codonopsis root), *shudi* (*Radix Rehmanniae Praeparata*, prepared rehmannia root), *maidong* (*Radix Ophiopogonis*, dwarf lilyturf tuber), *ejiao* (*Colla Corii Asini*, donkey-hide gelatin), *zhima* (*Semen Sesami Nigrum*, sesame), *fushen* (*Sclerotium Poriae Pararadicis*, Indian bread with hostwood), *suanzaoren* (*Semen Ziziphi Spinosae*, spiney date seed), *wuweizi* (*Fructus Schisandrae Chinensis*, Chinese magnolivine fruit), *muli* (*Concha Ostreae*, oyster shell), *fuxiaomai* (*Fructus Tritici Levis*, blighted wheat), and *nanzao* (*Fructus Jujubae*, Chinese date). (*Cheng Xingxuan's Case Records*)

◎证本液虚风动，舍滋水涵木，别无良策。（《斛山草堂医案》卷上）

（证候本是阴虚风动，除了滋水涵木，再没有别的办法了。）

The pattern is stirring of wind due to liver yin deficiency. Therefore, the only available choice is enriching water to moisten wood. There is no other solution. (*Case Records of Ganshan Cottage*) yìhuǒ bǔtǔ

益火补土

Replenishing Fire to Tonify Earth

通过温补肾阳以补助脾阳的治疗方法，又称为温肾健脾法、温补脾肾法、益火煖土法。根据五行与脏腑配属关系，心属火，脾属土，二脏为母子相生关系，益火补土当为温补心阳以补助脾土。但从命门学说兴起以来，此法嬗变为温补肾阳以暖脾阳的一种治法，用于肾阳衰微而致脾失健运之证，很少再指心火与脾阳的关系。代表方如四神丸、真武汤等。

The term refers to the therapeutic method of tonifying spleen yang by warming kidney yang, which is also known as fortifying spleen yang by warming kidney yang, warming and supplementing kidney-spleen yang, or replenishing fire to warm earth. According to the correspondence between the five elements and the zang-fu organs, the heart corresponds to fire, and the spleen corresponds to earth. As fire generates earth, there is a mother-child relationship between the heart and the spleen. Therefore, replenishing fire to tonify earth means warming and tonifying heart yang to assist spleen (earth) yang. However, the relationship between heart fire and spleen (earth) yang is rarely mentioned when the theory of *Mingmen* (命门, literally, gate of life) gains popularity. Instead, the method is developed into warming spleen yang by tonifying kidney yang which is applicable to the condition of the spleen failing to transport and transform due to kidney-yang debilitation. Representative formulas include *Sishen* Pill (Four-miracle Pill) and *Zhen Wu* Decoction (True Warrior Decoction).

【曾经译法】 supplement Fire for tonifying the Earth (Spleen)

【现行译法】 replenishing fire to generate earth (益火生土); replenishing fire to nourish earth

【标准译法】 replenishing fire to tonify earth

【翻译说明】 "益火补土"中"益"被译为 supplement 或 replenish；"补"被译为 tonify 或 nourish。"益""补"具体指温养火（肾）、土（脾胃）之阳，supplement 泛指补充，nourish 常指滋养、濡养，replenish 指补充使之重新充满，也可指添加燃料，如 to supply (a fire, stove, etc.) with fresh fuel。"补"选用 tonify，指补充、补益，常用于人体健康、医学领域。"益火补土"的内部逻辑关系为"益火"以"补土"，因此译为 replenishing fire to tonify earth。

引例 Citations:

◎夫少火为脾土之母，而实主运行三焦，熟腐五谷，故凡温中益火之剂，皆所以补其母也。(《内经知要》卷下)

（肾阳是脾土之母，而实际主宰运行三焦，腐熟五谷，所以凡是温中补阳的方剂，都是补其母。）

Kidney yang and spleen yang are of a mother-child relationship. Kidney yang is what governs the activities of triple energizer and the decomposition of food. Therefore, the composing of any formula to warm and tonify spleen yang follows the principle of supplementing mother organ to reinforce child organ (i.e., replenish fire to tonify earth). (*Essentials of the Internal Canon of Medicine*)

◎固以理脏真为最要，益火煖土，使下中之阳得安。(《评点叶案存真类编》卷上)

（原本以调理脏腑真气最为重要，益火补土，使中焦、下焦的阳气安宁。）

It is therefore of top priority to regulate authentic qi of the zang-fu organs. By replenishing fire (kidney yang) to tonify earth (spleen yang), yang qi in the middle energizer and the lower energizer will be harmonized. (*Classified Commentaries on Ye Gui's Medical Case Records*)

◎沙菀蒺藜茶……能温肾健脾，开胃进食，明目聪耳，益精壮阳。(《山居本草》卷四)

（沙菀蒺藜茶……有温肾健脾，开胃进食，明目聪耳，益精壮阳的功效。）

Shawanjili Tea (Flattened Milkvetch Seed Tea) ... can fortify spleen yang by warming kidney yang and improve appetite by strengthening the stomach. It also improves the health of eyes and ears as well as replenishes essence to improve sexual functions. (*Materia Medica Composed While Living in Mountain*)

金水相生

Mutual Generation Between Metal and Water

滋养肺肾阴液的治疗方法，又称滋养肺肾法。根据五行与脏腑配属关系，肺属金，肾属水，二脏为母子相生关系。当肺阴亏虚，不能滋养肾阴，或肾阴亏虚，不能滋养肺阴而致肺肾阴虚证时，治疗当同时滋养肺肾阴液，相互兼顾，使肺肾母子相生而获效。若金不生水，先有肺津亏虚，继而出现肾阴不足者，治宜补肺滋肾，方如百合固金汤。如果肾阴亏耗，虚火上炎，消烁肺津，当以滋肾为主，方如麦味地黄丸。

The term refers to the therapeutic method of nourishing yin fluids of the lung and the kidney, which is also known as enriching and nourishing both lung yin and kidney yin. According to the correspondence between the five elements and the zang-fu organs, the lung and the kidney correspond to metal and water respectively, with a mother-child relationship between them. Kidney-lung yin deficiency occurs when lung yin is deficient and fails to nourish kidney yin, or when kidney yin is deficient and fails to nourish lung yin. In this case, both lung yin and kidney yin should be enriched and nourished to promote their mutual generation for better therapeutic effects. Specifically, in the case of metal (lung) failing to generate water (kidney), with signs and symptoms of lung-fluid deficiency first and kidney-yin deficiency later, the main therapeutic method should be supplementing lung yin to nourish kidney yin. Formulae such as *Baihe Gujin* Decoction (Lily Bulb Metal-securing Decoction) are applicable. If the prominent cause is over-consumption of kidney yin leading to deficient kidney fire flaring up to consume the yin fluids of the lung, the main therapeutic method should be enriching kidney yin. Formulae such as *Mai Wei Dihuang* Pill (Dwarf Lilyturf Tuber, Schisandra and Rehmannia Pill) can be used.

【曾经译法】 generation between metal and water; mutual promotion between metal and water

【现行译法】 mutual promotion between lung and kidney; mutual promotion between metal and water; mutual generation between metal (lung) and water (kidney); mutual generation between metal and water

【标准译法】 mutual generation between metal and water

【翻译说明】 "相生"为五行生克的基本规律之一，被译为 mutual promotion, mutual generation。其中 mutual generation 为相对固定的术语翻译，也贴合"生"之本意。

引例 Citations:

◎端本澄源，仍不出六味合生脉，经岁常服，不特壮水制阳，兼得金水相生之妙用。(《古今医案按》卷二)

　　(从根本上加以调养，不外乎采用六味地黄丸配合生脉饮，常年服用，不仅可以滋阴制阳，还有金水相生的奇妙功效。)

To regulate and cultivate health by addressing the root cause, *Liuwei Dihuang Pill* (Six-ingredient Rehmannia Pill) in combination with *Shengmai* Drink (Pulse-activating Drink) should be taken throughout the year. Besides enriching yin to restrain yang, they work together to bring the miracle of mutual generation between metal and water. (*Commentaries on Ancient and Modern Case Records*)

◎如咳逆气短，甚则有汗，咽喉干燥者，当用金水相生法治之。(《时病论》卷七)

　　(如果咳嗽、气短，严重的伴有汗出，咽喉干燥，应当采用金水相生法治疗。)

For patients with cough, shortness of breath, or even sweating and dry throat in severe cases, the therapeutic method of mutual generation between metal and water should be adopted. (*Treatise on Seasonal Diseases*)

◎瘦人阴虚多火，六味地黄去泽泻合生脉散，使金水相生，自然火息痰降。（《张氏医通》卷九）

（形体消瘦的人阴虚多火，六味地黄去泽泻合生脉散，能使金水相生，自然火息痰降。）

Thin patients tend to have yin deficiency with hyperactive fire. For treatment, *Liuwei Dihuang Pill* (Six-ingredient Rehmannia Pill) minus *zexie* (*Rhizoma Alismatis*, alisma rhizome) in combination with *Shengmai* Drink (Pulse-activating Drink) should be used to promote mutual generation between metal and water, thus extinguishing fire and relieving phlegm. (*Comprehensive Medicine by Doctor Zhang Lu*)

三因制宜

Treating Diseases in Accordance with Three Factors

因时制宜、因地制宜、因人制宜的统称，是指临床治病要根据时令、地域、病人等具体情况，制定适宜的治疗方法。中医学认为人生活在大自然之中，自然界的各种因素必然会作用于人，同时，不同体质的个体也会做出不同的反应，产生不同的变化。因此疾病的发生、发展和转归与天时、地理以及人的体质等多重因素有十分密切的联系。所以，在治疗疾病时，除了重点考察症状、体征外，还必须进一步考虑其他多种因素，根据不同的情况，采取相宜的措施。三因制宜充分体现了中医学治病的整体观念，以及辨证论治过程中原则性与灵活性的有机结合。

The term refers to the principle of designing a suitable therapeutic method in accordance with particular seasonal and climatic factors, geographical environment, and the patient's specific condition. Traditional Chinese medicine (TCM) believes that people live in the natural environment and will undoubtedly be affected by various environmental factors. In addition, people may react differently to those influences and present different manifestations as their constitutions vary from person to person. Therefore, the onset, development, and progression of a disease are greatly affected by various factors, especially seasonal and climatic factors, geographical environment, and the patient's specific condition. In clinical practice, apart from analyzing signs and symptoms in detail, doctors should also take into consideration the above mentioned factors. Only through making a comprehensive analysis of all involved factors can a proper therapeutic method be determined. The concept of treating diseases in accordance with three factors not only embodies the holistic view, but reflects the integration of principle and flexibility in pattern differentiation in TCM.

【曾经译法】 treatment in accordance with three factors (season, locality and individual); triple pathogenies (三因)

【现行译法】 treatment of disease in accordance with three conditions; three categories of etiological factors (三因); three types of disease causes (三因); three types of etiologic factors (三因); three categories of disease cause (三因)

【标准译法】 treating diseases in accordance with three factors

【翻译说明】 "三因"之"因"被译为 factors, pathogenies, conditions, etiological factor 或 disease cause。由于"三因"指时令、地域、病人等具体情况，因此表示病因的词汇都过于具体，不够准确；factor 既可泛指，又可进一步指病因，较为合适。由于进一步解释"三因"会使术语过长，因此，不再具体翻译三个因素。

引例 Citations:

◎南方伤寒……挟暑宜正气散，挟寒宜五积散，此后贤因地制宜之说。（《医门棒喝》卷一）

　　（南方感受寒邪……夹暑邪的宜用正气散，夹寒邪的宜用五积散，
　　这就是后世医家因地制宜的观点。）

In the cases of cold damage in the southern area... if it is complicated with summer-heat, *Zhengqi* Powder (Qi-correcting Powder) should be used; if complicated with cold, *Wu Ji* Powder (Five Accumulations Powder) is more suitable. This illustrates the principle of treating diseases in accordance with geographical environment advanced by the doctors of later generations. (*Medical Warnings*)

◎乃于临证之顷，随病设施，揭其理蕴，而因时制宜，无法不备。（《医门棒喝·自序》）

（故在临证之时，根据病情治疗，阐明它的内在道理，根据时令采用适宜的治疗方法，则没有方法不具备。）

In clinical practice, one shall always find a solution if one could design a therapeutic method based on an analysis of the condition, understand its underlying rationale, and determine the treatment in accordance with the season and time. (*Medical Warnings*)

◎或药有因时、因人、因脉、因证之不同，总以治郁带补，清热宁嗽为吃紧耳。（《三合集》）

（或者用药有因为时令、病人、脉象、症状的差异，总体上以治疗郁滞兼以补益，清热止嗽为重要。）

The therapy may differ due to seasonal changes and differences in individual constitutions, pulse conditions, and other symptoms. Generally, the fundamental principle is to remove stagnation accompanied with tonification to relieve both heat and cough. (*Collective Case Records Conforming Pulse, Pattern, and Formula*) xuánhú jìshì

悬壶济世

Hanging Gourd to Help Patients

赞誉医生行医救人的事业。传说汉代时，河南一带出现了瘟疫，有许多人患病死去，当地的医生束手无策。一天，一个老人来到这里，他在一条巷子当中开了一家药店，门前挂上一个药葫芦，里面装着药丸，专治瘟疫。这位"壶翁"身怀绝技，乐善好施，只要有人求医，老人就会从药葫芦当中摸出一粒药丸，让患者以温开水服下。凡是喝了这位"壶翁"的药的人，病情都会很快好转。当时有个汝南人叫费长房，见这位老翁在人们离去后就跳入壶中，他觉得很奇怪，于是带上酒菜前去拜访，老翁便邀他一起进入壶中。费长房从此跟随他学道，壶翁把自己的"悬壶济世"之术教给他，共同行医。后人把此称为悬壶济世。

The term is used to praise life-saving professionals of traditional Chinese medicine. Legend has it that in the Han Dynasty, an epidemic disease attacked the area around Henan province. Many people died, but local doctors had no cure. One day, an old man came and he set up a medicine stand in a lane, hanging a gourd on the door. Stored in the gourd were some medicinal pills that could specifically treat the epidemic disease. With great skill and a kind heart, the old man would offer a pill to anyone who sought help from him and instruct the patient to take it with warm water. Anyone who took his medicine saw immediate effects. Fei Changfang, a native of Runan, observed that the old man would leap into the gourd after people left. Curiously, Fei paid a visit to the old man with prepared dishes and wine, and was then invited into the gourd. Since then, Fei was determined to learn skills from the old man, who taught all he knew to him. The two practiced medicine together. Hence, "hanging gourd to help patients" is used by later generations to refer to those who practice medicine.

【曾经译法】/

【现行译法】/

【标准译法】hanging gourd to help patients

【翻译说明】"悬壶济世"为中医行医治病的典型代名词，其中"壶"为葫芦，译为 gourd。"济世"实为挽救生命，因此建议意译，避免直译"济世"过于宏大，产生歧义。

引例 Citation:

◎费长房者，汝南人，曾为市掾。市中有老翁卖药，悬一壶于肆头，及市罢，辄跳入壶中，市人莫之见，唯长房于楼上睹之，异焉。（《后汉书·方术列传·费长房》）

（费长房，是汝南人，曾经是一个管理市场的官员。集市上有位行医卖药的老翁，他店铺前悬挂着一个葫芦，等到集市过午散去时，老翁便（化作一道烟，）钻进了葫芦内。集市上的人都没有看见过，只有费长房在楼上看到过，他心里感到十分惊奇。）

Fei Changfang was a native of Runan. At one time, he was a market administrator. There was an old man in the marketplace selling medicine at a stand with a gourd hanging in front. When the market was closed, he would (transform into smoke and) leap into the gourd. No one in the marketplace was ever able to see this, but Fei could from upstairs. He felt very curious. (*History of the Later Han Dynasty*)

神圣工巧

Miraculous, Sage, Skilled, and Ingenious

中医对望、闻、问、切四种诊断方法效果的称谓。出自《难经·六十一难》，认为通过望诊能够诊断疾病者为神奇，通过闻诊能够诊断疾病者为圣明，通过问诊能够诊断疾病者为工艺，通过切诊能够诊断疾病者为精巧。医生能四诊合参，就可达到神圣工巧的水平。

The term describes the four levels of expertise achieved by the doctors of traditional Chinese medicine through four respective diagnostic methods, namely, inspection, listening and smelling, inquiry, as well as pulse-taking and palpation. According to "The Sixty-first Issue" of *Canon of Difficult Issues*, having the ability to diagnose a disease through inspection is considered miraculous; through listening and smelling, sage; through inquiry, skilled; through pulse-taking and palpation, ingenious. By combining the four diagnostic methods, a doctor can achieve all four levels of expertise.

【曾经译法】 /

【现行译法】 /

【标准译法】 miraculous, sage, skilled, and ingenious

【翻译说明】 "神圣工巧"用于描述中医望闻问切四种诊断技艺的水平。其中"神""圣"偏重心智感官，分别译为 miraculous（奇迹般的；不可思议的）和 sage（睿智的，贤明的）。"工""巧"偏重技能程序，分别译为 skilled（熟练的；有技能的）和 ingenious（精巧的；巧妙的；有独创性的）。

引例 Citations:

◎经言望而知之谓之神，闻而知之谓之圣，问而知之谓之工，切脉而知之谓之巧。（《难经·六十一难》）

　　（医经上说，医生通过望诊能诊断疾病的称之为神，借助闻诊能诊断疾病的称之为圣，通过问诊能诊断疾病的称之为工，通过切脉能诊断疾病的称之为巧。）

According to medical classics, diagnosing a disease through inspection is considered miraculous; through listening and smelling, sage; through inquiry, skilled; through pulse-taking, ingenious. (*Canon of Difficult Issues*)

◎医不读《难》《素》，何以知神圣工巧，妙理奥义。（《三因极一病证方论》卷二）

　　（医生不读《难经》《素问》，怎么能知道神圣工巧，精微的道理和深奥的义理。）

Without reading *Canon of Difficult Issues* or *Plain Conversation,* how can a doctor understand the four levels of diagnostic expertise (miraculous, sage, skilled, and ingenious), the intricate theory, and the profound rationale? (*Discussion of Pathology Based on Triple Etiology Doctrine*)

◎望闻问切，神圣工巧，愚者昧之，明者了了。（《医经小学》卷二）

　　（望闻问切，神圣工巧，愚笨的人不明白，聪明的人懂得它。）

A fool will never understand the four examination methods (inspection, listening and smelling, inquiry, as well as pulse-taking and palpation) or the four corresponding levels of expertise (miraculous, sage, skilled, and ingenious), while a wise person savors them. (*Elementary Learning of Medical Canons*) jūnchénzuǒshǐ

君臣佐使

Monarch, Minister, Assistant, and Guide

中药方剂组织配伍的比拟词，君、臣本为古代治理国家的官职名称，分别在国家治理中发挥不同的作用，古代医家用以比喻处方中的主药和辅助药等。方剂一般由君药、臣药、佐药、使药四部分组成。其中君药是针对主病或主证起主要作用的药物，是方剂中必不可少的部分；臣药是辅助君药加强治疗作用或针对兼病或兼证的药物；佐药是协助君、臣药起治疗作用，或治疗次要兼证，或制约君、臣药的毒性与烈性，或为反佐药；使药是引导方中诸药直达病所，或调和诸药的药物。

The term illustrates metaphorically how a traditional Chinese medicine formula is composed. The "monarch" and the "minister" are officials in ancient China playing different roles in the governance of an empire. They are used to refer to the major medicinal and the assisting drug respectively. A formula is usually composed of monarch, minister, assistant, and guide medicinals. Among them, the monarch medicinal is the major one used to address the main disease or pattern, thus being indispensable in a formula. The minister medicinal is responsible for enhancing the effects of the monarch medicinal, or for addressing the accompanying disease or pattern. The assistant medicinal facilitates the monarch and the minister medicinals for better effects, treats minor symptoms, restrains the toxic or strong properties of the monarch and the minister medicinals, or works as the paradoxical assistant. The guide medicinal directs all medicinals toward the diseased site, or harmonizes all medicinals.

【曾经译法】 monarch, minister, assistant, and guide (indicating the different actions of medicines in a prescription); PRINCIPLES, ASSOCIATES, ADJUVENTS, AND MESSENGERS; monarch, minister, assistant, and guide; monarch, minister, adjuvant and dispatcher, key remedy and its adjuvants

【现行译法】monarch drug in a prescription (君药); ministerial drug (臣药); adjuvant drug (佐药); conductant drug (使药); sovereign [chief], minister [associate], adjuvant [assistant] and courier [guide]; monarch, minister, assistant and guide; monarch, minister, adjuvant and dispatcher; sovereign, minister, assistant and envoy; principal, subordinate, adjuvant, and guide; chief, deputy, assistant and envoy herbs

【标准译法】monarch, minister, assistant, and guide

【翻译说明】"君"被译为 monarch, principal, sovereign 或 chief。"臣"被译为 minister, associate, subordinate 或 deputy。"佐"被译为 assistant 或 adjuvant。"使"被译为 guide, messenger, dispatcher, courier 或 envoy。"君""臣"为古代官职名，因此保留其隐喻意，译为 monarch, minister。"佐"选用 assistant，延续"君臣"的拟人用法，而非 adjuvant（佐剂、佐药）。"使"主要表达"导引"之意，译为 guide。

引例 Citations:

◎主病之谓君，佐君之谓臣，应臣之谓使。(《素问·至真要大论》)
（主治疾病的就是君，辅佐君药的就是臣，附应臣药的就是使。）

In a formula, the key medicinal addressing the disease is called the monarch medicinal. The one that assists the monarch is the minister medicinal, and the one that coordinates with the minister medicinal is the guide medicinal. (*Plain Conversation*)

◎药有君臣佐使，大小奇偶之制。(《卫生宝鉴》卷三)
（药物有君、臣、佐、使，大方、小方、奇方、偶方的规定。）

A formula is usually composed of monarch, minister, assistant, and guide medicinals, and can be classified into a large, small, odd, or even one according to the numbers of included medicinals. (*Precious Mirror of Health*)

◎有君臣佐使之分，凡主病者为君而多，臣次之，佐又次之，须要察其兼见何症而佐使之。(《丹溪心法》卷十二)

> （药物有君、臣、佐、使的区分，凡主治疾病的就是君药而量多，臣药次之，佐药又次之，必须诊察他兼见什么症状而选用佐药与使药。）

In a formula, the medicinals are differentiated as monarch, minister, assistant, and guide. The monarch medicinal, greatest in quantity, serves the main function in treating the disease. The quantity of the minister medicinal is second to that of the monarch medicinal, and that of the assistant medicinal is even less. The assistant and guide medicinals are determined in accordance with the accompanying signs and symptoms. (*Danxi's Mastery of Medicine*)

四气五味

Four Qi and Five Flavors

四气五味又叫做"气味"或"性味"。这是中医用来说明中药作用的基本理论。中医学认为药物能治病的原因，主要是因为不同的药物具有不同的"气"和"味"，而不同的"气味"具有不同的治疗作用，所以用药物就可以对人体五脏六腑功能或器质上的各种病变，起到纠正和治疗作用。

四气又称"四性"，是指药物所具有的寒、热、温、凉四种性质。它是从药物作用于人体后，或者说是用以治疗疾病后所发生的效应所得出的一种药性的概括，凡能治疗热证的中药，大多属于寒性或凉性；凡能治疗寒证的中药，大多属于温性或热性。五味，是指药物有酸、苦、甘、辛、咸五种味道。五味不仅表示味觉感知的真实滋味，同时也反映药物的实际性能。中医学理论认为，食物或药物所具有的味，对人体分别有不同的作用。辛味能发汗解表、行气止痛，苦味能清热、解毒、泻火、燥湿，甘味能润补、缓急、和中，酸味能收敛、固涩，咸味能软坚散结、润肠通便。另外，五味之外，尚有淡味、涩味之说。

The term, also known as "qi and flavor" or "nature and flavor," refers to the fundamental theory used to explain the mechanism of traditional Chinese medicinals. With its own qi and flavor, a medicinal is believed to be able to treat specific patterns and will achieve its distinct therapeutic effects. Therefore, a combination of different medicinals can adjust and treat various pathological conditions of the zang-fu organs or organic lesions.

Four qi, also known as the "four natures," refers to the four properties of Chinese medicinals, i.e., cold, hot, warm, and cool. It summarizes the properties of medicinals based on their therapeutic effects. Specifically, medicinals for treating heat pattern mostly pertain to cold or cool natures, while those for cold pattern mostly pertain to hot or warm natures. The five flavors refer to sour, bitter, sweet, pungent, and salty tastes. They not only represent the flavors tasted by the tongue, but also reflect the actual functions of the medicinals. According to the theory of traditional Chinese medicine, different flavors of food or medicinals will exert varied effects on the human body. Specifically, the pungent flavor promotes sweating to release the exterior, and moves qi to relieve pain; the bitter flavor clears heat and fire, resolves toxin, purges fire, and dries dampness; the sweet flavor moistens, tonifies, relaxes spasm, and harmonizes the spleen and the stomach; the sour flavor astringes and consolidates; and the salty flavor softens hardness, dissipates masses, and moistens the intestines to promote defecation. Apart from the five flavors, there are also other flavors such as blandness and astringent flavor.

【曾经译法】 four natures of Chinese medicine (cold, hot, warm, and cool) (四气); FOUR PROPERTIES OF DRUGS (四气); FIVE TASTES OF DRUGS (五味); four characters (四气); five tastes (五味); the four natures (四气/性); five kinds of flavor (sour, bitter, sweet, pungent and salty) (五味); four properties of Herbs (四气); four natures of Herbs (四气); five kinds of flavor (sour, bitter, sweet, pungent and salty) (五味); four properties (四气)

【现行译法】 five kinds of tastes (五味); four natures (四气); five tastes (flavors) (五味); four properties and five tastes; four properties and five flavors of herbs; four nature of drugs (四气); five flavours (五味); four qi (四气); five flavors (五味); four properties (四气)

【标准译法】 four qi and five flavors

【翻译说明】 "四气"之"气"被译为 nature, property, character 或 qi；"五味"之"味"被译为 taste 或 flavor。"五味"之"味"，虽既指口味，又指药物功效，但术语无法兼顾，优先表达"口味"之意较妥。由于 flavor 较 taste 词义更为单纯，因此选用。

引例 Citations:

◎药有酸咸甘苦辛五味，又有寒热温凉四气，及有毒无毒。（《神农本草经》卷一）

（药物有酸、咸、甘、苦、辛五种味道，又有寒、热、温、凉四种性质，以及有毒、无毒的不同。）

Medicinals differ in flavor (sour, salty, sweet, bitter, and pungent) and qi (cold, hot, warm, and cool). They may also differ regarding being toxic or nontoxic. (*Agriculture God's Canon of Materia Medica*)

◎味有五，气有四，五味之中各有四气。（《本草纲目》卷一）

（味道有五种，气性有四种，而五味之中又各有寒热温凉四性。）

The medicinals have five flavors and four qi/natures. For each of the five flavors, it may have the nature of cold, hot, warm or cool. (*Compendium of Materia Medica*)

◎若药具五味，备四气，君臣佐使配合得宜，岂有此害哉？（《本草纲目》卷十四）

（如果药物具有五味、四气的特性，君臣佐使配伍得当，怎么能有这样的灾害呢？）

How can malpractice occur if one can accurately differentiate the flavor and qi of each medicinal, and compose the formula in accordance with the principle of properly combining monarch, minister, assistant, and guide medicinals? (*Compendium of Materia Medica*)

升降浮沉

Ascending, Descending, Floating, and Sinking

　　升降浮沉是表示药物作用趋向的一种性能，是药物作用的定向理论。一般而言，升，即上升提举，表示药物作用趋向于上；降，即下达降逆，表示药物作用趋向于下；浮，即向外发散，表示药物作用趋向于外；沉，即向内敛藏，表示药物作用趋向于内。升降浮沉分别表示药物向上、向下、向外、向内四种不同的作用趋向，是与疾病所表现的趋向性相对而言的。其中，升与降，浮与沉是相对立的，而升与浮，沉与降，既有区别，又有交叉，难以截然分开，在实际应用中，升与浮，沉与降常并称。按阴阳属性区分，则升浮属阳，沉降属阴。

　　中药的趋向性作用，主要是通过药物作用于机体后所产生的功能效应而概括出来的。大凡药物能针对病变部位在上在表或病势下陷发挥治疗作用者，其作用趋向多确定为升浮；凡药物能针对病变部位在下在里或病势上逆发挥治疗作用者，其作用趋向多确定为沉降。一般而言，升浮药主上升向外，有升阳、发表、散寒、涌吐、开窍等功效；沉降药主下行向内，有潜阳、降逆、泻下、利水、收敛等功效。

The term, as a concept of drug action, is used to describe the direction-related tendencies of pharmacological effects of Chinese medicinals. Generally, *sheng* (升, ascending) indicates the upward movement to lift; *jiang* (降, descending), the downward movement to downbear; *fu* (浮, floating), moving toward the exterior to diffuse; *chen* (沉, sinking), moving toward the interior to store. Ascending, descending, floating, and sinking represent respectively the upward, downward, outward, and inward movement of medicinal effects and are contrary to the tendency of the disease. They can be classified into two pairs, namely, ascending versus descending and floating versus sinking. For each pair, they are different yet overlapping, which makes it difficult to clearly tell them apart. In clinical practice, ascending and floating are often combined, so are descending and sinking. In terms of yin-yang property, ascending and floating pertain to yang, while descending and sinking pertain to yin.

The tendencies of pharmacological effects of Chinese medicinals are inferred according to their effects on the human body. For the medicinals effective in treating diseases in the upper or exterior part or relieving sinking tendency/ manifestations, they are labeled as ascending and floating; for those effective in treating diseases in the lower or interior part or directing adverse flow of qi downward, they are labeled as descending and sinking. Generally, ascending and floating medicinals, with the tendency to move upward and outward, work to lift yang, release the exterior, dissipate cold, induce vomiting, and open the orifices, etc.; descending and sinking medicinals, with the tendency to move downward and inward, work to subdue hyperactive yang, direct the counterflow of qi downward, purge, promote urination, and astringe, etc.

【曾经译法】 lift, lower, float, sink (referring to action of Chinese materia medica); lifting, lowering, floating, sinking; ascending, descending, floating, sinking; ascending, descending, floating and sinking

【现行译法】 lifting, lowering, floating, sinking; ascending, descending, floating and sinking; upbearing, downbearing, floating and sinking; ascending and descending, floating and sinking; upbearing, downbearing, floating and sinking

【标准译法】 ascending, descending, floating, and sinking

【翻译说明】 "升降浮沉"主要表示药物的作用趋向，因此选用明确表示方向趋向性的词汇，更为契合术语含义。按照约定俗成原则，译为 ascending, descending, floating, and sinking。

引例 Citations:

◎升降浮沉：凡药，轻虚者浮而升，重实者沉而降。(《素仙简要》)
　　(升降浮沉：凡药物性质轻而空虚的浮而升，重而中实的沉而降。)

Ascending, descending, floating, and sinking: a medicinal that is light and hollow tends to float and ascend, while one that is heavy and solid tends to sink and descend. (*Concise Medicinal Principles of Suxian*)

◎药推寒热温凉平和之气，辛甘淡苦酸咸之味，升降浮沉之性，宣通泻补之能。（《仁斋直指方》卷一）

> （用药应推论其寒、热、温、凉、平的性质，辛、甘、淡、苦、酸、咸的味道，升降、浮沉的作用趋向，宣发、疏通、补益、泻下的功效。）

When prescribing medicines, one should judge whether a medicinal is cold, hot, warm, cool, or neutral, whether its flavor is pungent, sweet, bland, bitter, sour, or salty, whether its moving tendency is ascending, descending, floating, or sinking, and whether it works to diffuse, unblock, tonify, or purge. (*Renzhai's Direct Guidance on Formulas*)

◎盖甘之味有升降浮沉，可上可下，可内可外，有和有缓，有补有泻，居中之道尽矣。（《汤液本草》卷中）

> （甘味有升降、浮沉的作用趋向，可以上升，也可以下降，可以向内，也可以向外，既调和又缓急，既补益又攻泻，完全居于中庸之道。）

The sweet flavor fits the golden mean: sweet medicinals can not only ascend, descend, float, and sink, but also harmonize, relieve spasm, tonify, and purge. (*Materia Medica for Decoctions*)

术语表 List of Concepts

索引 Index
(按音序 In Chinese Alphabetical Order)

参考文献 References

1. Wong K. Chimin (王吉民) & Wu Lien-Teh (伍连德). *History of Chinese Medicine*. Shanghai: National Quarantine Service. 1936

2. 广州中医学院《汉英常用中医词汇》编写组. 汉英常用中医词汇. 广州: 广东科技出版社. 1982

3. 帅学忠. 汉英双解常用中医名词术语. 长沙: 湖南科技出版社. 1983

4. 欧明. 汉英中医辞典. 广州: 广东科技出版社. 三联书店香港分店. 1986

5. Paul U. Unschuld. *Nan-Jing*. California: University of California Press. 1986

6. 汉英、汉法、汉德、汉日、汉俄医学大词典编纂委员会. 汉英医学大词典. 北京: 人民卫生出版社. 1987

7. Cheng Xinnong (程莘农). *Chinese Acupuncture and Moxibustion*. Beijing: Foreign Languages Press. 1987

8. Dan Bensky & Randall Barolet. *Chinese Herbal Medicine: Formulas & Strategies*. Washington: Eastland Press. 1990

9. 李照国. 中医翻译导论. 西安: 西北大学出版社. 1993

10. 刘占文. 汉英中医药学词典. 北京: 中医古籍出版社. 1994

11. Nigel Wiseman（魏迺杰）. 英汉汉英中医词典. 长沙: 湖南科学技术出版社. 1995

12. 黄嘉陵. 最新汉英中医词典. 成都: 四川辞书出版社. 1997

13. 李照国. 中医英语翻译技巧. 北京: 人民卫生出版社. 1997

14. 石学敏, 张孟辰. 汉英双解针灸大辞典. 北京: 华夏出版社. 1998

15. 张奇文主编, 孙衡山译. 实用汉英中医词典. 济南: 山东科学技术出版社. 2001

16. 李照国. 简明汉英中医词典. 上海: 上海科学技术出版社. 2002

17. 谢竹藩. 新编汉英中医药分类词典. 北京: 外文出版社. 2002

18. Nigel Wiseman & Feng Ye. *A Practical Dictionary of Chinese Medicine*. 北京: 人民卫生出版社. 2002

19. 方廷钰, 陈锋, 王梦琼. 新汉英中医学词典. 北京: 中国医药科技出版社. 2003

20. 谢竹藩. 中医药常用名词术语英译. 北京: 中国中医药出版社. 2004

21. 全国科学技术名词审定委员会. 中医药学名词. 北京: 科学出版社. 2005

22. World Health Organization Western Pacific Region. *WHO International Standard Terminologies on Traditional Medicine in the Western Pacific Region*. Manila: Philippines. 2007

23. 李振吉. 中医基本名词术语中英对照国际标准. 北京: 人民卫生出版社. 2008

24. 李照国. 简明汉英黄帝内经词典. 北京: 人民卫生出版社. 2011

25. 方廷钰, 嵇波, 吴青. 新汉英中医学词典（第 2 版）. 北京: 中国医药科技出版社. 2013

26. 李照国. 汉英双解中医临床标准术语辞典. 上海: 上海科学技术出版社. 2016

中国历史年代简表 A Brief Chronology of Chinese History

远古时代 Prehistory			
夏 Xia Dynasty			c. 2070 - 1600 BC
商 Shang Dynasty			1600 - 1046 BC
周 Zhou Dynasty	西周 Western Zhou Dynasty		1046 - 771 BC
	东周 Eastern Zhou Dynasty 春秋时代 Spring and Autumn Period 战国时代 Warring States Period		770 - 256 BC 770 - 476 BC 475 - 221 BC
秦 Qin Dynasty			221 - 206 BC
汉 Han Dynasty	西汉 Western Han Dynasty		206 BC-AD 25
	东汉 Eastern Han Dynasty		25 - 220
三国 Three Kingdoms	魏 Kingdom of Wei		220 - 265
	蜀 Kingdom of Shu		221 - 263
	吴 Kingdom of Wu		222 - 280
晋 Jin Dynasty	西晋 Western Jin Dynasty		265 - 317
	东晋 Eastern Jin Dynasty 十六国 Sixteen States*		317 - 420 304 - 439
南北朝 Southern and Northern Dynasties	南朝 Southern Dynasties	宋 Song Dynasty	420 - 479
		齐 Qi Dynasty	479 - 502
		梁 Liang Dynasty	502 - 557
		陈 Chen Dynasty	557 - 589
	北朝 Northern Dynasties	北魏 Northern Wei Dynasty	386 - 534
		东魏 Eastern Wei Dynasty 北齐 Northern Qi Dynasty	534 - 550 550 - 577
		西魏 Western Wei Dynasty 北周 Northern Zhou Dynasty	535 - 556 557 - 581

隋 Sui Dynasty		581 - 618
唐 Tang Dynasty		618 - 907
五代十国 Five Dynasties and Ten States	后梁 Later Liang Dynasty	907 - 923
	后唐 Later Tang Dynasty	923 - 936
	后晋 Later Jin Dynasty	936 - 947
	后汉 Later Han Dynasty	947 - 950
	后周 Later Zhou Dynasty	951 - 960
	十国 Ten States**	902 - 979
宋 Song Dynasty	北宋 Northern Song Dynasty	960 - 1127
	南宋 Southern Song Dynasty	1127 - 1279
辽 Liao Dynasty		907 - 1125
西夏 Western Xia Dynasty		1038 - 1227
金 Jin Dynasty		1115 - 1234
元 Yuan Dynasty		1206 - 1368
明 Ming Dynasty		1368 - 1644
清 Qing Dynasty		1616 - 1911
中华民国 Republic of China		1912 - 1949

中华人民共和国1949年10月1日成立
People's Republic of China, founded on October 1, 1949

*"十六国"指东晋时期在我国北方等地建立的十六个地方割据政权，包括：汉（前赵）、成（成汉）、前凉、后赵（魏）、前燕、前秦、后燕、后秦、西秦、后凉、南凉、南燕、西凉、北凉、北燕、夏。

The "Sixteen States" refers to a series of local regimes established in the northern area and other regions of China during the Eastern Jin Dynasty, including Han (Former Zhao), Cheng (Cheng Han), Former Liang, Later Zhao (Wei), Former Yan, Former Qin, Later Yan, Later Qin, Western Qin, Later Liang, Southern Liang, Southern Yan, Western Liang, Northern Liang, Northern Yan, and Xia.

**"十国"指五代时期先后存在的十个地方割据政权，包括：吴、前蜀、吴越、楚、闽、南汉、荆南（南平）、后蜀、南唐、北汉。

The "Ten States" refers to the ten local regimes established during the Five Dynasties period, including Wu, Former Shu, Wuyue, Chu, Min, Southern Han, Jingnan (also Nanping), Later Shu, Southern Tang, and Northern Han.